ADVANCE PRAISE

"*Healing and Cancer* is a must read for both patients with cancer and their practitioners as a guide to optimizing both the care and caring of the whole person facing one of life's greatest challenges. Kudos to Jonas and McManamon for truly putting patients first!"

—Leonard H. Calabrese, DO, Professor of Medicine, CCLCM, R.J. Fasenmyer Chair in Clinical Immunology, Theodore F. Classen Chair in Osteopathic Research and Education, Rheumatic and Immunologic Diseases, Cleveland Clinic

"*Healing and Cancer* creates a road map for clinicians to ensure they are keeping the patient, and what is important to them, at the front and center of their cancer treatment. It lays out how to do whole person care in an often fast-paced and under-resourced environment. Every cancer clinician should have a copy of this book and make it a part of how they provide care."

—Jennifer Bires, MSW, LCSW, OSW-C, CST, Executive Director, Life With Cancer and Patient Experience, Inova Schar Cancer Institute

"This guide is equally pertinent for patients, caregivers, and healthcare professionals, underscoring the vital role of embracing and enacting whole person care in reshaping our healthcare system and enhancing the well-being of our society."

—Lorenzo Cohen, PhD, Professor and Director, Integrative Medicine Program, MD Anderson Cancer Center and co-author of *Anticancer Living: Transform Your Life and Health with the Mix of Six*

"If you or someone you loved were facing a diagnosis of cancer, the care described in this text is what you would aspire to receive. An excellent resource that should be read by all with cancer or who care for those with cancer!"

—Mary Jo Kreitzer PhD, RN, FAAN, FNAP, Chair for Health and Wellbeing Leadership, Director, Earl E. Bakken Center for Spirituality & Healing

". . . [W]ith experience and insight honed by years of clinical leadership, the authors poignantly illustrate a golden rule of medicine—'healing is a whole person affair, the product of each individual's unique biology, social circumstances, and personal goals'—and they point us all in the direction health care needs to change to the benefit of patients, families, clinicians, health care organizations, and policymakers alike."

—Michael McGinnis, MD, MA, MPP, Leonard D. Schaeffer Executive Officer and Senior Scholar, National Academy of Medicine

"This is a brilliant book, describing the way cancer care should be for everyone. If you or a loved one has cancer, buy this book, and give it to your oncologist and your oncology team. Highly recommended."

—Dean Ornish, MD, Founder & President, Preventive Medicine Research Institute, Clinical Professor of Medicine, University of California, San Francisco

"Patients with cancer as well as their family and friends would be well served by reading the *Healing and Cancer* guidebook written by Wayne Jonas and Alyssa McManamon, who have broad experience as innovators in the field of cancer."

—Debu Tripathy, MD, Professor and Chair, Department of Breast Medical Oncology, The University of Texas MD Anderson Cancer Center

"This is a landmark book that I consider essential reading for people with cancer and all those caring for them. Drs. Jonas and McManamon provide us with a comprehensive overview of the science and application of whole-person care, as well as practical tools and resources that care teams can use now to improve the quality and length of life of cancer patients."

—Andrew Weil, MD, Lovell-Jones Professor of Integrative Medicine

"I highly recommend this book to anyone who has cancer and everyone supporting them, especially their medical team. It is a *must have resource* for all cancer centers and oncology clinics/ units of every institution."

—Daniel Vicario, M.D., ABIHM, Co-Founder,
Board Member, Director Integrative Oncology,
San Diego Cancer Research Institute

Healing and Cancer is an invaluable resource for promoting patient activation in their care. With a focus shifted from 'what's the matter' to 'what matters,' whole person cancer care increases our sensitivity to the real needs of the person living with cancer. The resources and tools provided in this guidebook will facilitate the ability of cancer care givers to better meet the needs of our patients and provide them with the whole person cancer care they so fervently desire and deserve."

—Donald I. Abrams, MD, Integrative Oncology,
UCSF Osher Center for Integrative Health

"The book *Healing and Cancer* by Drs. Jonas and McManamon sets a new standard for high-quality cancer care. It is a must read for any healthcare practitioner interacting with cancer patients. While modern oncology has made tremendous strides in changing cancer from a death sentence to a chronic disease, the holistic approach outlined in this book points to the next giant step in cancer care."

—Emeran A. Mayer, MD, Director, G. Oppenheimer Center for
Neurobiology of Stress & Resilience, UCLA Vatche & Tamar
Manoukian Division of Digestive Diseases, UCLA

"Healing and Cancer, by Drs. Wayne Jonas and Alyssa McManamon, is an enlightening arms-wide-open embrace of the rapidly expanding universe of evidence and opportunities for whole person cancer care. This is a truly marvelous work that, in a world where so much feels disjointed and disconnected, offers hope by uniting patients and practitioners in a shared purpose—healing."

—Steve Bierman, MD Author, Healing Beyond Pills and Potions, Board Certified Emergency Physician at Scripps Memorial Hospital

"In *Healing and Cancer* the authors provide us a much needed integrative and holistic approach to cancer that addresses the needs of the mind, body and spirit."

—VADM(Ret) Richard Carmona, MD, MPH, FACS, 17th Surgeon General of The United States

"Healing and Cancer sheds light on blending evidence-informed cancer care and whole-person care that is 'both/and' not either/or.' This whole person approach helps patients to live more intentionally and to access their inner resources of strengths and clarity for what matters most. This is a jewel of a book."

—Barbara Dossey, PhD, RN, FAAN, author of,
Florence Nightingale: Mystic, Visionary, Healer
and Holistic Nursing: A Handbook for Practice

"Drs. Jonas and McManamon provide a much-needed blueprint for how health systems can embrace the whole oncology patient. Kudos for their work!"

—Heather Greenlee, ND, PhD, Medical Director, Integrative Medicine, Director, Cook for Your Life (cookforyourlife.org), Fred Hutchinson Cancer Center

"Written by pioneering physicians, *Healing and Cancer,* is a magnificent contribution in caring for people living with serious illness within their values and life story. It is a brilliant synthesis for everything that is needed to transform the crisis of cancer, hopelessness, and helplessness into strength and wisdom. This book is destined to become a classic."

"In this groundbreaking work, Drs. Jonas and McManamon expertly articulate a compelling vision for the key components of Whole Person Care. More importantly, they outline a clear pathway to make the vision into a reality. I strongly recommend this book for all those affected by cancer."

"We go into medicine to care for the *whole person*. This book not only reminds us of our calling, it gives us the tools to do so more effectively."

"*Healing and Cancer* is a beautiful, loving and helpful guide to caring for people with cancer and for caring about people with cancer. Oncology teams will recognize themselves and the work they do in the expert, experienced and open approach the authors take to complex care across the continuum of cancer diagnosis, treatment and recovery, with equally helpful insight when curing is not possible and caring continues. *Healing and Cancer* is an essential reference for practicing and training providers of all disciplines.

"You have heard of the 'Moon Shot' in cancer? Now here is the 'Moon Landing'! It is a must-read book from a prominent researcher and clinician for anyone involved in cancer care or healing from cancer . . . this is the book that you need."

—Kenneth R. Pelletier, PhD, MD, Clinical Professor of Medicine
(UCSF Med), Author of *Change Your Genes, Change Your Life*

"This beautifully written and profoundly wise book about the practice of a medicine of the whole person in the setting of cancer is a gift to everyone who feels disempowered when cure is not possible. *Healing and Cancer* reminds us all that healing exists in the absence of cure and offers us proven and highly innovative approaches to evoke it."

—Rachel Naomi Remen, MD, author of
Kitchen Table Wisdom, My Grandfather's Blessings

"The rapid development of precision medicine and immunotherapy as new strategies for treating cancer will only reach their full potential in the context of comprehensive whole person care. *Healing and Cancer* is a must-read for all healthcare professionals devoted to improving the lives of people living with cancer."

—Ray Wadlow, MD, Medical Oncologist,
Inova Schar Cancer Institute

HEALING
AND CANCER

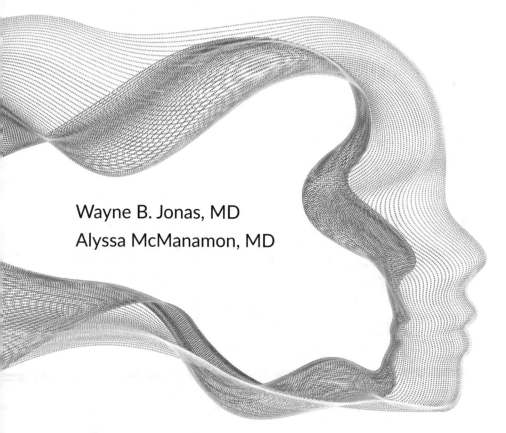

Wayne B. Jonas, MD
Alyssa McManamon, MD

A Guide to
WHOLE PERSON CARE

RODIN
BOOKS™

Hardcover ISBN 978-1-957588-24-7
eBook ISBN 978-1-957588-25-4

PUBLISHED BY RODIN BOOKS INC.
666 Old Country Road
Suite 510
Garden City, New York 11530

www.rodinbooks.com
Cover design by Six Half Dozen
Book design by Alexia Garaventa

Manufactured in the United States of America

RODIN
BOOKS.

Dr Wayne Jonas
To my wife, Susan C. Jonas, without whom both this book and "what matters" to me in life would not exist.

Dr Alyssa McManamon
To the ones who ask, "Where is the patient voice?"

CONTENTS

ABBREVIATIONS—ACRONYMS

ACS American Cancer Society

AHRQ Agency for Healthcare Research and Quality

AI artificial intelligence

ASCO American Society of Clinical Oncology

CBD cannabidiol

CDC Centers for Disease Control

CMS Centers for Medicare & Medicaid Services

EHR electronic health record

EMT emergency medical technician

FDA Food and Drug Administration

HIPAA Health Insurance Portability and Accountability Act

ICU intensive care unit

LDL low density lipids

NCCN National Comprehensive Cancer Network

NCI National Cancer Institute

NIH National Institutes of Health

NSAID nonsteroidal anti-inflammatory drugs

PSA prostate-specific antigen

PTSD post-traumatic stress disorder

SIO Society for Integrative Oncology

THC tetrahydrocannabinol

VA Veterans Health Administration

WHO World Health Organization

PREFACE

The purpose of this book is to bring the concepts of healing and whole person care further into oncology and health care so that people diagnosed with cancer feel better and live longer. Oncology teams want to manage the fear and confusion that comes along with the disease. They want to bring the full science of cancer biology into the care of the patient. They want time and better tools to help the person with cancer into full engagement in their own care and address what matters most.

When care teams do this, they establish the highest quality of care for people with cancer and for themselves.

We all need to spend more time doing this because too often cancer care today does not consider the whole person. Most cancer care focuses on killing the cancer cell and in the process supports a major industry to do that, more and better. While this is a laudable goal, it drives an imbalance in the type of care people receive. This creates a situation wherein clinical teams are caught on a treadmill not of their own making, with ever-increasing demands on their time for tasks that may not directly impact the health, healing, and survival of their patients.

Such a narrow focus has great costs. For the person, there are costs in time, money, side effects, suffering, and fear. For the team, there are costs in the joy of practice, the energy to improve health care delivery, and in their overall vitality and burnout. Often, the needs of patients who those on the team see and know should be addressed, are pushed to the background for lack of time, tools, and money. Moral injury ensues.

A pivot to healing over curing is often found at the end of a cancer journey, when the shadow of the cancer cell no longer obscures the other needs of a person—needs that were there all along but could not be addressed. Care teams know how to address these needs. Although not easy in our current system, we suggest a pivot to whole person care is possible for all people with cancer, to the degree that their diagnosis, personal values, and their care teams' capabilities allow. Oncology teams who practice deep listening to patients *as people* and are given the time and resources can move beyond patient-centered care to what we call person-centered or whole person care. With increasing numbers of people surviving cancer and the intensity and duration of relationships in oncology, we suggest this is a field uniquely positioned to further the uptake of whole person care happening throughout medicine.

In this book we will define whole person cancer care and illustrate how this type of care can become standard in all of oncology. We summarize the science behind whole person care and the evidence that supports its application. We bring in examples of how it's being done from small clinics to large institutions. Finally, the book points readers to the best tools and resources available that oncologists, cancer care teams, and people with cancer can incorporate into their own healing journey.

Who should read this book? Our hope is that this book will be read and actively used by health care leaders, by teams caring for people with cancer, by caregivers, and by patients themselves. Readers will learn how the science of whole person care can be implemented both to treat cancer and to enhance wellbeing and longer life.

The book has 3 parts.

Part One describes what whole person care and healing are and the rationale behind them. We summarize the evidence behind whole person cancer care and describe how the patient, family, friends, and the wider care community can be successful in using that science more effectively. We show the reader some simple tools to help them enhance wellbeing for themselves and for patients.

Part Two will take the reader through the stages experienced along the cancer journey, from being diagnosed with cancer, through treatment, to the end of treatment, and after. We use examples of usual cancer care to illustrate what happens, and then show what *can* happen to optimize healing at each stage of the journey. We describe frameworks and models of practice used in the VA and other hospitals in the US and globally, and how they are working to embed whole person care into their systems.

Part Three provides resources that any system or practice leader, oncologist and care team, including nurses, social workers, administrators, medical assistants, and others can use to optimize cancer care. These tools and resources have been selected from multiple sources including professional guidelines, published research, vetted websites, and experts in whole person care. They are drawn from tested tools in general medicine and then modified for use in cancer by a group of more than 20 oncology leaders during bimonthly meetings held over 2 years. For care teams working to make whole person care routine and regular, we point to additional credible and regularly updated sources of information and ideas for practice improvement.

How to use this book. This book and its supplemental resources are designed to improve the care of people with cancer. We recommend that Part One of the book be read through as a whole. It provides the *why* and *what* of whole person care. For readers in positions to make change in a practice environment and ready to do so, a read of Part Two gives ideas on *where* and *when* to implement changes. It describes places along the cancer journey where these changes can be made. Part Three provides tools and resources for making selected changes, as desired, whether at the micro or macro levels. We address how to optimize individual wellbeing as well as examples of how systems have changed to improve whole person care in oncology, despite the complexity of cancer care. We point to simple tools that can be used now and describe approaches to changemaking throughout the book. The book website (www.HealingandCancerBook.com) highlights additional resources for practice change, tips for team engagement, and a workbook to help organize change.

While we draw from extensive evidence and experience, it is not any team's or individual's knowledge alone that allows for healing. Instead, it is the sensemaking we all bring to the complexity of cancer, our acknowledgement of the emotions surrounding it, and the uniqueness of any one human being's experience. Whole person care puts the person with cancer and their wisdom first—their history and circumstance, their intuition, their knowledge of self and body, their understanding of what makes for a good life and a good death. We offer this information with humility and suggest that we all thrive when whole person care is a reality.

Let's get started.

AUTHORS' NOTES

DR WAYNE JONAS

Science tells us that cancer is a disease of cells. But it's really a disease of people. Whole people—and their loved ones. When my wife first got cancer, she was 36 years old, and we had 3 young children. We quickly learned just how the diagnosis affects mind, body, and spirit. How its effects spread to friends and colleagues, communities, and countries. How it generates fear and focus. How it influences the perception of our shared future. How it confronts us with death and forces us to face and often find what is most important in life. To find what matters most. And better ways to heal.

Since then, I have cared for patients with cancer, both as their primary care doctor before and after the diagnosis, and as a consultant for many cancer patients under the care of oncology teams. I have, like most physicians, seen patients who refused conventional care die; some who only did conventional care die. I have also seen similar patients in both categories stay alive and thrive. In all cases, patients and their care teams needed the time and tools to look wider than they usually did, and help in making decisions that best fit everyone's needs. Some conversations were gentle and guiding. Some were frank and difficult.

In all cases, what works best is to bring in the science, hold out realistic hope, and guide people toward decisions where they feel comfortable and empowered. In my practice, I aim to hold a space for healing always, curing sometimes, with patience and compassion as often as I can.

DR ALYSSA MCMANAMON

A piece of advice for medical students: Go into a residency training where you like the people, or at least where you are like the people. The OBGYNs liked me, but I wasn't feeling it (sorry—one particular program in the '90s). I enjoyed mutual admiration with family physicians, but I had yet to spend a month with 4 hematology-oncology doctors. Two I liked, and 2 were puzzling (one chain-smoked outside the clinic). I recall most about the one who rounded late, after clinic. We sat (or rather, he sat and I stood behind him) for what felt like (and was) hours. At any bedside meeting, he barely spoke at first. Listening to the patient with his eyes shut, his head shook or nodded, only rarely mumbling, "Mmmhmm." I had never seen a doctor listen so intently. Patients loved him.

Recently, I viewed an introduction video posted by his practice. In it, he said all the things he taught me by example more than 30 years ago. With a brief mention of how much we receive from our patients, he began:

> First, discuss with the patients what they understand of their disease, as this can change. Second, make sure a patient can see what you see and understand. Third, understand the goals of the patient—what they really want. As he pointed out, "Not everyone wants the same thing." Fourth, lay out the options for treatment and draw the patient in to understand the risks and benefits and how those might support their goals. Fifth, make sure they know we always have ways we can help, no

matter how bad the disease. Sixth, let them know that this practice isn't just an office, but a very caring and empathetic place, where you are treated like family.

His gift of listening was also for those of us who stood silently behind him, learning from him, over hours and hours of priceless time. I am here because listening matters.

THE INTEGRATIVE ONCOLOGY LEADERSHIP COLLABORATIVE

We often heard calls from other physicians, nurses, and teams working with people who had cancer that more information and tools were needed to deliver whole person care in routine practice. We decided to pull together a leadership group of oncology teams to help build those tools and processes. Called the Integrative Oncology Leadership Collaborative (IOLC), the group adapted successful whole person care models and methods from primary care for use in oncology. This book is drawn from that 2-year collaborative, our personal practice and research experience of over 60 combined years, and the latest science on what works and why for healing and cancer.

Our cancer care system is dysfunctional, making whole person care difficult. But the people in it are some of the most caring, compassionate, and knowledgeable people who exist, all seeking the best for treatment of disease and alleviation of suffering. It is for them this book is written.

A NOTE ON PATIENT STORIES AND PRIVACY

The clinical cases described in this book are drawn from our practices. We have compressed or edited them for reasons of clarity and brevity. To honor the privacy of each person, names and some details may have been changed to protect those who wish to remain anonymous.

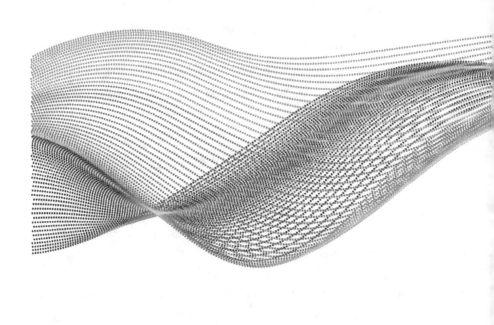

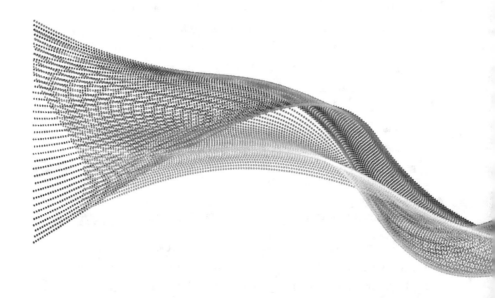

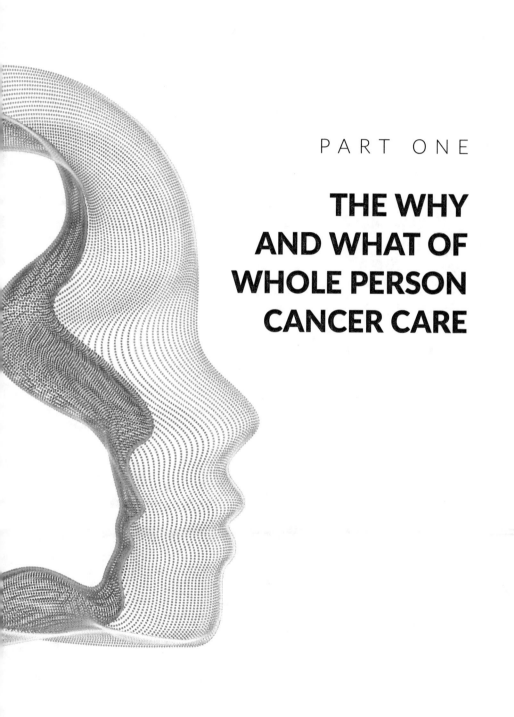

PART ONE

THE WHY AND WHAT OF WHOLE PERSON CANCER CARE

CHAPTER ONE

CANCER INVOLVES THE WHOLE PERSON

When all systems are working well, a person with cancer can actively heal. Like a computer program running in the background, healing of the person is a process occurring all the time. Teams that work to support and enhance this inherent healing capacity find that their patients not only do better and feel better, but they can also live longer. Oncology teams and others who work with patients to achieve better outcomes may even find more satisfaction in their work. The purpose of this chapter is to demonstrate how we can learn to see our patients as whole people—not just their disease—and help them to use the best clinical medicine along with the full range of effective social and mental health practices, supportive and palliative care, lifestyle and self-care, and complementary and integrative treatments. We will introduce a patient we refer to throughout the book, an actual patient who has, over decades, faced a life with cancer. We call her Jan. But first, we start by defining and describing what whole person care is.

WHAT IS A WHOLE PERSON?

What is a whole person? To do whole person care requires us to know what that means. In the modern era one of the most accepted and durable models of human flourishing is Maslow's Hierarchy of Needs. The following figure illustrates the model as developed by the American psychologist over 70 years ago.

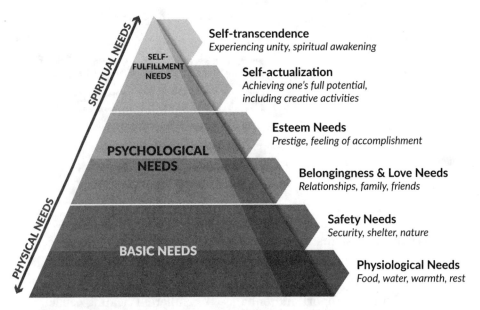

Figure 1.1 Maslow's Updated Hierarchy of Needs

Maslow arranged these from basic, physical needs at the bottom, through security and safety needs, to social and psychological fulfillment, to spiritual needs at the top. Our reorganization of these needs acknowledges that they are basic requirements for human flourishing and provide the basis for seeing a whole person and operationalizing whole person care.

At the bottom of the hierarchy are basic physical needs—food, water, shelter, safety. In the middle are psychological and social needs—relationships, family, love, esteem. At the top are self-fulfillment needs—creativity, self-actualization, and the experience of unity and joy in life. Maslow hypothesized that we start with the basic needs and then a healthy individual gradually moves up the hierarchy to self-transcendence. These are what all humans need to flourish.

However, since Maslow's time, we have discovered several things about human flourishing. First, these factors are not in a strict hierarchy. Some people can draw on social support and spiritual strength even without their basic needs being met. Some people with basic needs totally fulfilled still drift without purpose. Individuals flourish when all areas are adequately addressed. When people are seen from only one aspect, care is not whole person.

To accommodate these more recent shifts in knowledge and understanding, and to operationalize a whole person model of human wellbeing in health care, we have created the HOPE model. HOPE stands for Healing-Oriented Practices and Environments, and places the domains of Maslow's hierarchy into a set of concentric circles containing the elements of Maslow's pyramid but organized in a way that enhances the ability to see and work with people as whole people, multilayered and complex.

On the outside are the physical aspects of a person—the areas of body and physical place. Then comes the behavioral aspects of who we are; factors that we now know are major contributors to health and wellness—healthy food, movement, sleep, relaxation. Then there are the deeper and less visible domains of a person—first, the social and emotional dimensions, and then, at the center, the mental and spiritual dimensions. It is these 2 deeper domains that are often neglected in medicine and health care. It is the last dimension—mental and spiritual—that most often brings forward what most deeply matters to a person. Each of these dimensions are essential to consider when caring for ourselves or others. Throughout this book we will return repeatedly to this framework of a whole person, using it to help organize how we can care for a person with cancer. We will use the story of Jan, a person who experienced several cancers over many years to illustrate both the challenges and successes of whole person care.

Body & External

Behavior & Lifestyle

Social & Emotional

Spiritual & Mental

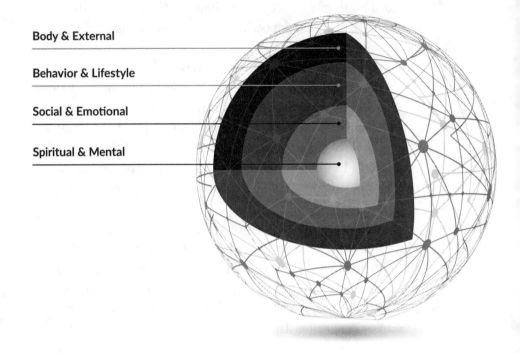

Figure 1.2 What Is a Whole Person?

This reorganization of the domains of what a whole person is, helps us see the operationalized care for the whole person. The outside layers of the physical person are the easiest to see and care for. As we look for and perceive the deeper layers of a person, the dimensions, while not as visible, are just as real and essential to human health and wellbeing as the outside.

INTRODUCING JAN

Year after year, Jan returns to her childhood home in the lush, green forests of South Florida. She walks by the water in the canals, the lakes, and the ocean. Her family moved from the north when she was a baby, and she grew up here as a young child and teenager before going off to college and a whole new world. Still, she comes back every year—to see her family, the water, the sky, how the plants have grown, and the landscape changed. She looks for what's the same, as well as what's different.

It was in Florida that she lived through the joys and traumas of her childhood, learned lifestyle habits, and walked barefoot in the streets and on the beach, her pale Irish skin exposed to the hot Florida sun. It is here where she was exposed to pesticides as they sprayed the mosquitoes, and it was here where she was buffeted by the stresses of growing up poor. Here she learned the resilience she would need in the future—the resilience to compartmentalize and to adapt.

At first, things didn't seem to change in Florida on her trips back. Rains came down. Clouds drifted by. The ocean and the sky remained the same. But then new buildings and roads began to spring up as easily as the plants grew up in the warm sun. The land was still beautiful and green, but an impending threat was already in place. Invasive plant species were entering South Florida and pushing out the native species. Like a cancer on the land, they were taking over and growing in an uncontrolled manner, sucking up the nutrients and the water.

Then, a threat emerged in her own body. At 34, with 2 young children, the first cancer arrived—triple negative breast cancer in a premenopausal woman. The prognosis for a young woman like her was statistically not good, but she adapted. After surgery, chemotherapy, and radiation, followed by an experimental vaccine, she was cancer-free.

She changed her career from accountant to counselor. She volunteered in her community, spent more time with her kids, and joined their school's leadership. Twenty-five years went by as the world's understanding of cancer advanced, but Jan didn't know about those advances. She didn't need to.

Then, like the invasive species growing in her childhood home, the cancers started coming back at increasingly shorter intervals. Melanoma appeared on her back in 2008, treated with surgery. A second one on her scalp 5 years later. Then, a second type of breast cancer in 2016, on the same side as the first, likely induced from the radiation for her first cancer. This one was treated with surgery and chemotherapy again, followed by an aromatase inhibitor.

Two years later, ovarian cancer was found during prophylactic surgery. It had already spread to her abdomen. She was treated again with surgery and chemotherapy—an even harsher combination this time. That's when her oncologist tested for and discovered the BARD-1 gene variant, a risk for both breast and ovarian cancer, but not a mutation that has a treatment. In 2022, the ovarian cancer spread again, prompting more surgery and more chemo.

Now, as she walks among the gardens in South Florida, the cancer grows inside her again. In the Everglades, simply poisoning and pulling out invasive species is not enough. Environmentalists also need to plant and cultivate a diverse ecological system that can help to better control the rogue species. They need to support the health of the environment in ways that will keep all the native species strong.

A BIGGER TOOLBOX

Jan now needs more tools than her regular oncology team can offer. She needs a wider lens, one that can focus on her as a whole person. She needs something to support her wellbeing and personal ecology, something that will crowd out the cancer cells, or at least slow them down, without poisoning and stripping the rest of her body. Science knows what needs to go into those tools and teams, but the full set of tools is not easily accessible, not easily seen, and not usually integrated into regular cancer care.

We know, for example, that eating a wide variety of plant foods and fiber will nourish a healthy gut microbiome and help the immune system to control cancer. But does her gut work enough while on chemo to benefit from such a diet? We know that certain herbs and safer drugs can change the drivers of cancer progression. But we don't know what doses or combinations to use, and how to personalize them to each patient. We know we need to talk about cancer like any other chronic disease, as a disease with ups and downs to be managed. Cancer is there long before we see it and may come back long after we thought we killed it. It is an invasive species that is, strangely, of our own body.

That view is hard to hold when the massive cancer industry talks almost entirely about "breakthroughs," "moonshots," and the "war" to "cure." Those words and the systems it spawns keep us from seeing the true nature of the disease. Do we have a magic cure for any other chronic disease, such as obesity, diabetes, heart disease, or Alzheimer's disease? Why do we believe cancer is different? Why do we fail to see it as a chronic disease to be managed holistically, rather than only rogue cells to be killed?

When we take a broader view of treatment, however, we see tools such as diet, exercise, mind-body practices, and social support for wellness as essential, not simply nice to have. These approaches are safe, but they will never reach the type and level of evidence required for, say, FDA approval of a drug. They can't be patented, so they make no money and get little research investment. At least not enough to drive the 16 years and $1 billion typically invested to bring a new drug to market.[1]

In addition, there are the tools of complementary medicine: safe treatments that fall outside the mainstream of conventional medicine. Valuable as they are when used with conventional treatments, they are rarely taught in medical training or paid for by insurance. While integrative medicine brings conventional and complementary approaches together to treat the whole person and not just the cancer, it is still not the mainstream approach. Even though we have evidence that even minimal access to whole person care can improve and possibly lengthen the lifespan for people with cancer, it's not surprising that not 1 person on any of Jan's oncology teams, over nearly 30 years and multiple cancers, ever mentioned these complementary tools.[2]

Jan accepted the conventional treatments her oncology team had to offer, but decided to look beyond them for tools that would do more than kill cancer cells. She needed tools that would heal her and improve her quality of life. Her oncology team had little guidance to offer. Jan was on her own to find those tools, evaluate them, access them—and pay for them. She had no map to guide her into whole person care. Fortunately for Jan, she had access to family and friends with strong ties to the integrative medicine community.

They were able to guide her to safe complementary treatments and skilled providers who understood her condition and her goals. She has access to more tools in a bigger medical bag than before—something all people with cancer should have, but don't.

THE SCIENCE OF WHOLE PERSON CARE

The war on cancer and the "cancer moonshot" may not have achieved their goals yet, but one thing they have done is provide us with an abundance of research demonstrating the need for a whole person approach to the prevention and treatment of cancer. Extensive evidence now demonstrates that cancer cells arise within an environment—both a microenvironment in the tissues surrounding the cancer, and a macroenvironment of the person's body as a whole. The micro, macro, and environmental exposures we all have are as important for the development and disappearance of cancer as killing the cancer cells.

This realization has resulted in radically different treatment approaches than the cut, burn, and poison of past oncology practices. One such innovation involves manipulation of the immune system to identify and control the cancer. Immunotherapy treatments, such as the drug pembrolizumab (Keytruda®), remove a shield that protects some cancers from being detected and removed by the immune system. This science has also resulted in new vaccines that in some cases completely prevent cancer, such as the HPV vaccine for preventing human papilloma virus-associated cancers, such as cervical, throat, and anal cancers. Once harnessed, the immune system is able to do its job and dutifully eliminates the rogue cells. Another major innovation involves manipulating the nutrition and metabolism of the cancer cell environment. Newer therapies, such as vascular endothelial growth factor (VEGF) inhibitors block the growth of blood vessels that feed cancer cells and inhibit the cancer's use of glucose or other energy sources, including oxygen. A third new area is the systematic targeting of cancer drivers, or what are called the "hallmarks of cancer."[3] These are factors that cancers often exploit to keep growing and spreading. They either drive or inhibit a cancer's progression, metastasis, or regression. This has generated a whole series of new drugs under the umbrella term "precision oncology."

NO MAGIC BULLETS

Magic bullets have proven elusive, despite an extensive search for them. Billions of dollars, both public and private, have streamed into these new areas of cancer treatment. And while there have been a few exceptional examples of dramatic regressions, these approaches have for the most part occurred in only a small minority of patients whose tumors meet very specific target requirements. Even when patients have these drivers, many of the new drugs targeting them don't work. Since 2000, the FDA has approved more than 92 drugs for solid tumors. Only a handful have displaced existing first-line drugs. The new drugs have on average resulted in only 2.8 months of life extension.[4] This minimal achievement comes at great cost in quality of life, side effects, and money.

The biology of cancer shows us why. Cancer is not a single disease, but an evolving and complex mixture of tumor types, even within the same tumor and the same person. This all occurs within the ecological network of interactions we call the environment of the whole person. It only makes sense that, like the poisoning of invasive species in Jan's Florida, trying to hit single targets with single drugs cannot, by its very nature, have large effects for most people. What is needed are broad-based interventions that involve the whole tumor environment and the whole person, in all their complexity. Unfortunately, cancer-industry investments, research support, and practice guidelines are all structured to test and recommend only one treatment at a time. They haven't focused on possible safe combinations and person-driven approaches that might control and manage the disease throughout its trajectory.

There are no magic bullets. Yet our system is designed to keep looking for them and delivering what we find on a silver platter, one at a time. And, of course, patients want a magic bullet, too. The science says that for most people, this is a false hope.

WHOLE PERSON CARE

What is the alternative? For the Jans of the world and those who care for them, the answer is obvious: Whole person care. Such a system of care uses the best conventional and complementary treatments, but also pays attention to the biopsychosocial and spiritual nature of life with this disease, and to the environment and context in which the person and the cancer live.

We have discussed Maslow's hierarchy as a model of human flourishing. At first, the top of his hierarchy was "self-actualization." But toward the end of his life, Maslow added the spiritual needs of a person seeking self-transcendence, resulting in greater happiness and wisdom. A cancer diagnosis is a challenge to all these needs simultaneously, making them crystal clear. Because research has significantly advanced our knowledge of what produces wellbeing and a flourishing life, we can update and enhance Maslow's hierarchy. We now know that it is not just food that keeps people healthy, but the content and amount of food people need for optimal health. We know the ideal activity level and types. We know the importance of stress management and addressing trauma. And we have tools for improving our mental and spiritual health and wellbeing. We know not only what those needs are, but better ways to fulfill them. (We summarize this evidence in Chapters 4 and 5.)

We also know that healing and wellbeing are not strictly hierarchical, to be approached like a checklist starting at the bottom, and only later addressing the top. Human flourishing and healing require that our care addresses all the components, in almost any order. There are multiple pathways to healing. Individuals without optimal physical circumstances can still find great wellbeing through social and spiritual support. And many with ideal social and spiritual support could still improve their nutrition and activity. What we need is a way to address all aspects of human flourishing and wellbeing from the beginning through the end of life. We need a system for whole person care.

This is the *raison d'être* and the challenge of whole person cancer care. We need to help people along their healing journey while seeing cancer for what it is, whether an immediate life threat or a chronic condition to be managed throughout life. Whole person care involves being honest and comprehensive about the evidence we have and don't have, being more careful about words like "cure," and providing real hope, even in the midst of complexity and uncertainty. Few people like Jan have 5 different cancers over 35 years. But few people are "one and done" when they get cancer either. The diagnosis leaves a trace, if not a gaping hole to fill. Let's work, even amid a broken system, to help all people receive such healing throughout their lives.

THE CURRENT SYSTEM SUCKS

Whether you are an oncologist, advanced practice provider, nurse, medical assistant, navigator, social worker, or any other cancer team member, or if you're a person with cancer or a caregiver, you're likely to agree that the current system for managing cancer sucks.

Care is now so complex we need teams to provide it, and we need navigators to guide people along the way. People are thankful to receive holistic care but entwined are also logistical frustrations, time toxicity, financial stress, and even dehumanizing experiences. The narrow regulatory environment and pharmaceutical company drivers force the search for single-agent treatments and limit our tools largely to expensive drugs. The volume of patients required in any practice to make ends meet drive a burnout treadmill. The logistics of coordinating appointments, tests, information access across various systems, lab work (including the growing number of genetic and genomic tests recommended), treatment approvals by insurance companies, transportation, and time management are a nightmare. The costs of treatment and the lack of coverage lead to financial toxicity and bankruptcy. Cancer care teams don't have the time and tools to fully explain the benefits and risks of various options in plain, understandable, and accurate language.

And all these challenges are just around trying to deal with the tumor! Things become even more complicated when we decide to care for the whole person. We all want people with cancer to have less fear, fewer side effects, easier access to care, and a longer life. Everyone in the system has the patients' best interests in mind. Cancer care teams and the vast cancer industry are made up of good people trapped in dysfunctional systems. Our goal with this book is to give you sufficient inspiration and information so that your cancer care team and patients can move toward more whole person care even in the system we have and, hopefully, by doing so, change it for the better.

THE GOOD NEWS

Despite the immense system challenges, examples of whole person care are breaking out all over. Whole person care approaches in the US and abroad are discussed in the recent National Academy of Medicine (NAM) report, *Achieving Whole Health*.[5] Requested by the VA and cosponsored by the VA, the Samueli Foundation, and the Whole Health Institute, the first part of the report is a detailed look at the extensive evidence for whole person care and examples of that type of care happening around the world. Almost all systems moving toward whole person care have shown improvement in the quadruple aims all health care shares, including:

1. Patients doing better and having better satisfaction

2. Reducing costs

3. Improving access, equity, and population health

4. Improving the work life of health care providers, helping them be happier and reducing burnout[6]

Recently, an additional aim—equity—has been added to the recommended core outcomes.[7]

In 2021, Dr Jonas and his team developed an Integrative Healthcare Learning Collaborative (IHLC) network made up of 16 primary care practices around the country. These practices used a simple set of tools and resources, called the Healing Oriented Practices and Environments (HOPE) Note Toolkit, to organize their visits around whole person care. These tools and how they have been modified for cancer care from primary care are described in Chapter 11. Many health systems have now incorporated these tools and processes into their routine visits. CMS has gradually attempted to create advanced payment models in primary care to encourage and support these practices. And the NAM has completed an additional study exploring how adjustments in health care payments, purchasing, and investment money could scale and spread these practices.[8]

WHOLE PERSON CANCER CARE MODELS

Whole person care models have also been picked up by leaders in oncology. In 2013, the National Academy of Medicine published a comprehensive study of person-centered care in cancer. Called *Delivering High-Quality Cancer Care,* the study summarized the evidence, gave examples, and made recommendations on how to implement this type of care around the country.[9]

Building on that report, CMS released 2 rounds of bundled payment approaches. The first, in 2016, was the Oncology Care Model, designed to encourage innovations in these approaches.[10] Nearly 200 oncology practices or systems signed up and implemented efforts to enhance whole person care. This has been followed by another funding program called the Enhancing Oncology Model, which seeks to build on these approaches. In parallel with this, the world's largest cancer professional organization, ASCO, along with the Community Oncology Alliance (COA), developed a certification program for practices implementing the Oncology Medical Home (OMH), another model moving toward whole person cancer care. Nine programs have achieved that certification. We need more.

These models seek to integrate the multiple services provided at many cancer centers for whole person care into more organized delivery. This integration often includes services such as psycho-oncology, integrative oncology, lifestyle resources, supportive care, palliative care, social work, financial support, spiritual care, patient navigation and advocacy, shared decision-making, survivorship, and others.

HOPE FOR CANCER

In 2021, the authors of this book organized a network of oncology leaders from around the world, called the Integrative Oncology Leadership Collaborative (IOLC), to adapt the HOPE tools and resources being applied in primary care for use in oncology. These tools are designed specifically to help organize and implement the extensive resources available for whole person care more effectively into oncology practices and systems. These tools include the Personal Health Inventory (PHI), adapted from the VA; the HOPE Note Toolkit, used to guide the cancer team's discussion and planning with patients; and the Personal Healing Plan (PHP), a set of action items that reflects the joint goals of person and providers organized through shared decision-making. In addition, we have collected numerous resources for use by oncology teams and patients to help them understand and apply whole person care in routine practice. Finally, we described a framework (The Two-Circle Model for Whole Person Care) being used by health systems to help them reengineer their quality improvement approaches for better integration of whole person care in cancer management.

A growing number of cancer practices and systems are using various strategies to provide whole person care from the time of first diagnosis, through treatment, to recovery, or the end of life.

Our hope for those reading this book is that, despite the system challenges, we can all move forward in small steps toward whole person care in our practices. This is happening increasingly both nationally and around the world—it's possible for you and your team as well.

SUMMARY POINTS

- Cancer impacts the whole person, not just individual cells.
- Healing in the person and evolution of the cancer occur simultaneously. Whole person care means we treat the cancer and support the healing of the person simultaneously.
- Whole people are made up of a physical body and external

dimensions, their behavior and lifestyle, their social and emotional dimensions, and their mental and spiritual aspects.

- The science of cancer now shows that the environment of the whole person around the cancer significantly influences the behavior of the cancer.

- There are major challenges to whole person cancer care built into our current systems.

- The HOPE Note Toolkit (HOPE standing for Healing-Oriented Practices and Environments) applied in primary care are now available for use in cancer care.

- This book is a guide for teams on how to implement whole person care in oncology.

CHAPTER TWO

ENGAGING THE PERSON IN CANCER CARE

We know from the science of cancer biology that cancer is not, like an infection or accident, something that happens to you. It *is* you—an aberration to be sure, but still the result of your cells going rogue and your body and immune system unable to control them. We also know that on a largely invisible and microscopic level, cancer cells constantly evolve—progress and regress. They are influenced by viruses and vaccines, smoking, alcohol and diet, environmental toxins, activity and stress, and other internal and external factors. All of this occurs within a whole person and many of these factors are influenced by behavior and the environment—social, psychological, and physical.

Once the cancer becomes visible, however, the way we usually approach it largely ignores these whole person factors. Instead, we focus on trying to shrink it using surgery, drugs, and radiation. The process almost immediately disempowers a person from being actively involved in a care plan. The language is technical and confusing; teams look to avoid any hint of blame for the person; the surgical, medical, and radiation oncologists focus on their craft to stay at the top of their game in treatment, and the cancer industry pushes its latest drug or technology to kill the cell. All this basically says to the person with cancer, "Hang tight, we're coming to rescue you," and an uneven power dynamic is immediately established.

One of the most challenging aspects of whole person care is changing this message and process so that the patient and their co-survivors become active participants in their own care, and a key part of their own team. In this chapter, we talk about ways to help make that happen and the benefits of doing so.

THE BIDIRECTIONAL NATURE OF HEALING

In accepting help, let alone being rescued, we realize we may incur a debt of sorts. In facing cancer, a person may feel there's no choice about accepting help. It's like a car accident: someone is going to call for help, even if it's not us. In cancer medicine today, most patients feel they can't help themselves—things are done to them and for them, and their role is simply to follow instructions. To accept help in a way that allows treatment to work best for both the person with cancer and the care team, we all need to feel safe enough to ask questions, safe enough to admit we don't know everything, safe enough to let our guards down, and to determine when and what we will do together.

Physician-author Rachel Naomi Remen said it best: "Helping incurs debt. When you help someone, they owe you one. But serving, like healing, is mutual. There is no debt. I am as served as the person I am serving. When I help, I have a feeling of satisfaction. When I serve, I have a feeling of gratitude. These are very different things." Dr Remen ends her essay, "From the perspective of service, we are all connected: All suffering is like my suffering, and all joy is like my joy. The impulse to serve emerges naturally and inevitably from this way of seeing. Lastly, fixing and helping are the basis of curing but not of healing. In 40 years of chronic illness, I have been helped by many people and fixed by a great many others who did not see my wholeness. All that fixing and helping left me wounded in some important and fundamental ways. Expertise cures, but only service heals."[1]

One of the most important lessons Dr Jonas learned about healing occurred before he started medical school. He recalls:

> I was doing a rotation in a hospital as a student chaplain and was assigned to minister to a man dying of advanced cancer. He was on a morphine pump and seemed to be sleeping as I entered the room and sat next to him. I was young and nervous, uncertain how to minister to this person, many decades my senior. So, I closed my eyes and started to pray for him. A few minutes later I felt his hand touch my hand, which startled me. I opened my eyes. There he was, looking directly at me and smiling. "Thank you for coming, son," he said gently. "You're going to be all right." Our roles were instantly reversed. In picking up on my nervousness and despite his pain and suffering, he was healing me! As Rachel Remen said, healing is mutual, with reciprocal benefit, if we will open our eyes and see it.

When Jan got her third recurrence of ovarian cancer, a new oncologist who was fresh off a prestigious fellowship training took over her treatment. Based on the doctor's training pedigree, he was one of the best in the world, but had little experience in the nuances of patient needs and individual responses to treatment. After several mishaps with chemotherapy doses, Jan took the initiative. She knew her body and its responses and she ended up guiding the oncology care team to better management. The best expert on the patient is . . . the patient. We need to accept that as real and spend the time to get to know the person with cancer.

GETTING TO ENGAGEMENT

Every year, some 2 million Americans are told they have cancer. The diagnosis often arrives as a thunderbolt, upending their lives—and the lives of those around them. When people encounter the oncology care team for the first time, they're often in a state of shock—fearful and confused. They're deluged with unfamiliar terminology about cancer and its treatment while also dealing with a storm of emotions and concerns for the future. This moment, when people may feel they have stepped over a cliff, is the time to begin engaging the person and those around them in whole person care. From the beginning, the team can acknowledge and begin to address fear and anxiety. The team can let them know that they have work to do between visits—they need to learn about their own role in treatment and recovery beyond worrying. As an example of a "healing assignment," the patient and family can be asked to identify their cancer care advocate, or read an article on self-care, or explore any recommended integrative complementary therapies that will support their healing, such as acupuncture or yoga (see Chapter 12 for resources patients can access). The team can also set up a time for a HOPE or whole person care visit, as we'll discuss in Chapter 11. This process can be established simply, with the oncologist mentioning that they like for patients to engage in "healing work" (or some other active term) between visits and that the social worker, nurse, or medical assistant will provide that assignment with related resources. This then goes on the next steps and follow-up list at checkout and follow up.

Bringing the person into their own cancer care and facilitating, after first acknowledging, their inherent healing capacity or wholeness, is the first step in implementing whole person care. To do this, we need to know them as more than a person with cancer—we need to know their biology, their psychology, their lifestyle, their environment, their social situation, and their meaning and purpose in life. We need to listen to them to know what matters to them as a person. From there, we invite them and the people around them, gently or directly, depending on the circumstance, to be an integral part of the care team. As we start to build rapport, one early step (after acknowledging them as whole people) is to gain clarity on who this person wants to be the boss moving forward. Most typically, people with cancer quickly say they want the expertise of our team to be the boss. Even when we're the designated boss, however, the care team can make it clear that the patient is really the ultimate boss and can stop the process at any point. We can pull from the 3 Ws of patient safety and teach patients that it's OK to say:

1. What you see

2. What you're concerned about

3. What you want to have happen

We can also teach patients and caregivers the "Stop the Line" process used by high-reliability organizations, like the VA, to avoid harm when a potential problem is identified. This framing can help patients know up front that you want and need their active involvement in their care.

The collective expertise of cancer care teams means they can be intimidating to patients. The power differential can close off open communication. To avoid that, we need to give explicit permission (or at least open the opportunity) for people to speak up at any time for any reason. The 3 Ws are an easy way to get that across—and studies back it up.[2] Most care settings lack a clear structure for patients and families to speak out and "Stop the Line" if necessary. This presents an opportunity for quality improvement in oncology practice. If you're a care team member and have taken safety training such as the AHRQ Team STEPPS, you have some tools to draw from. Share them with patients in a meaningful way, such as putting up posters showing the CUS statements from the training: "I am Concerned! I am Uncomfortable! This is a Safety issue!" Consider if or how your practice allows patients and families a voice in real-time quality improvement. If it's missing, you have a next step to get to patient engagement for your practice. Infusion nurses have frequent opportunities to reinforce and empower people during chemotherapy. While checking and double-checking dose and patient identification, taking a few minutes to double check with the patient on any symptom or life goal needs communicates that safety involves everyone.

GUIDANCE TO GET THERE

The Institute of Medicine (IOM, now the National Academy of Medicine), in its report *Delivering High-Quality Cancer Care,* considers engaged patients "central to an effective, efficient, and continuously learning system."[3] They recommend some steps oncology practices can take to meet patient engagement goals:

- Improving decision aids and making them available through print, electronic, and social media
- Providing professional educational programs for members of the cancer care team that include comprehensive and formal training in communication
- Improving communication with patients with advanced cancer
- Ensuring members of the cancer care team receive education and formal training in end-of-life communication
- Evaluating and potentially improving the current process for handling advance care plans
- Evaluating and potentially improving the current process for providing palliative care, psychosocial support, and timely referral to hospice care for end-of-life care

These recommendations (and others provided in this book and its website) are a good framework for an oncology practice to deliver several components of whole person care. A big part of communication is active listening. Modern aspects of busy training programs and practice mean we may find ourselves unable to listen enough to learn, whether from a trainer or our patients. Check out continuing education offerings from places like the Institute for Healthcare Communication (healthcarecomm.org). None of us is born knowing how to communicate optimally. It's an acquired skill.

Engaging the person with cancer means sharing power and responsibility, with information flowing in both directions and with the person as an active partner in making decisions. When our teams do this well, the benefits are mutual. Figure 2.1 shows

"The 5Ts for Teach Back," a patient engagement tool to enhance information delivery and reception.

People engaged in their own care are more motivated to:

- Take steps to improve their health
- Make values-driven decisions that further healing
- Keep appointments and ask questions
- Feel satisfied with their care

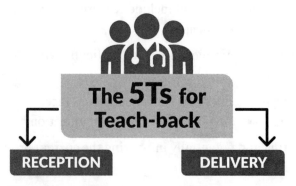

RECEPTION

Take Responsibility:
"I want to make sure I did a good job explaining..."

Tell Me:
Ask the patient to tell you, in their own words, what they will do or what they understand. Be explicit about what you want the patient to say back.

DELIVERY

Triage:
Focus on just one topic for teach back.

Tools:
Use a model, a written tool, a poster, graphics, etc. to help you explain what you want your patient to know.

Try Again:
If necessary.

Figure 2.1 Communication Tool: The Five Ts for Teach Back

Adapted from Anderson KM, Leister S, De Rego R. The 5Ts for Teach Back: An operational definition for teach-back training. Health Lit Res Pract. *2020;4(2):e94-e103. It is designed to enhance listening and communication and improve the mutual understanding of what was discussed between patient and clinical team.*

The IOM's report gives a good starting point, with 2 specific recommendations. First, from the very beginning the cancer care team can provide patients and their families with clear, understandable information on:

- Their particular cancer and prognosis
- Treatment benefits and potential harm
- Types of palliative care
- Types of psychosocial support
- Estimates of the total and out-of-pocket costs of their care

Note that with the advance of information sources such as "Dr Google" and AI engines, honing skills in how to help patients use those resources wisely is especially important. ASCO's Cancer.Net has reliable patient education on the topic of evaluating cancer information on the internet and includes a 5-minute video of an oncologist speaking on how to identify cancer misinformation. Viewing this safe site could be the "assignment" you give a patient and allows for a shared mental model in care planning (while acting as an invitation to discuss what they find online).

The second IOM recommendation applies for people with advanced cancer: Provide people with end-of-life care consistent with their needs, values, and preferences. The care team can only know these, of course, if they are engaged with the person from the beginning (see also Chapter 10 discussing end-of-life issues). In whole person care, we can add an additional recommendation: Provide clear, understandable information on the value of taking an active, integrative approach to care. Then be prepared to offer resources that are timely, trusted, and meet their stated needs, whether to control symptoms, improve wellbeing, or reduce risk of recurrence. Care teams can only learn of patients' needs, values, and preferences by asking. The asking is followed by listening and sharing people's responses for all on the care team to see and know. This process can be helped by having succinct information sources and aids to facilitate more complex decisions.

DECISION AND DIALOGUE AIDS

Decision aids, often in the form of questions to ask your health care provider, are valuable tools for helping people with cancer make informed, values-based choices about their treatment. Decision aids help patients navigate the pros and cons of treatment options and come to good decisions based on accurate information combined with their personal values and their individual situations.[4] Written materials, such as web-based decision aids and pamphlets, may not be as helpful for those with low health literacy, as they often require an eighth grade reading level and technology access. Patients who are open to tech use at an appropriate level of literacy can be directed to free apps such as Cancer.Net, which contains informative articles, videos, podcasts, and other media and has tools for organizing appointment schedules, tracking side effects, and keeping lists of questions for the care team. We provide links to further resources throughout Part Three of this book, this book's website www.HealingandCancerBook.com, and on the Healing Works Foundation website (www.healingworks-foundation.org).

Our patients face complex decisions every day, such as deciding on reconstructive surgery after a mastectomy and what kind, or whether early prostate cancer needs to be treated and if so, how? We're there to assist because these decisions can be challenging to make, but we're not available around the clock. Decision aids have the potential to reduce anxiety and give people the knowledge they need to participate fully in making an informed choice. They're designed to help patients see the potential outcomes of their decisions at each point—along with the alternatives—and know what questions to ask the care team. From the care team's perspective, decision aids have the potential to improve communication, assure that the decisions are made with the person's input and perspective, reduce decisional conflict, and lead to personalized choices based on accurate information. They can potentially lead people to better satisfaction with their decision and a more realistic understanding of the possible outcomes of treatment.[5,6]

If your team recommends decision aids or uses them regularly, also consider tools that help people think about the future beyond cancer treatment. For integrative cancer care planning at younger ages, Healing Works Foundation created, with professional and patient input, a whole person-based tool called My Treatment, My Life (offered in 2 versions, as Cancer Choices for Young Adults 23-29 years old and Cancer Choices for Teens and New Adults 15-22 years old). They're found on the Healing Works Foundation website (www. healingworksfoundation.org) and landing page for this book.

Those websites also have information on how to help patients navigate the many complementary and integrative medicine (CIM) recommendations they will come across. Since most cancer patients investigate and use these approaches, knowing how to discuss and navigate this information is an important part of whole person care for the oncology team.

In Chapter 11, we discuss a number of tools that are useful for starting and maintaining dialogue with patients about "what matters" for them. One of those tools is the Personal Health Inventory (PHI), originally developed in the VA as part of their approach to care, Whole Health, and subsequently adapted for use in general primary care and oncology. It takes only a few minutes for patients to fill out before a visit and can rapidly start a dialogue about social, emotional, behavioral, and wellness factors important for their care. When incorporated into a visit designed to specifically discuss this with the person and link them to whole person resources provided in Part Three of this book, an ongoing dialogue to help maintain patient engagement and empowerment becomes regular and routine.

SHARED DECISION-MAKING

ASCO's annual meeting in Chicago in 2023 brought over 40,000 attendees together (in person and virtually) to learn how to better care for people with cancer. The meeting's theme was "Partnering with Patients: The Cornerstone of Cancer Care and Research." The Presidential Address was given by Dr Eric Winer, esteemed clinician-researcher, and Director of the Yale Cancer Center, in

New Haven, Connecticut. He spoke candidly of his personal experience as a patient with hemophilia and HIV. We listened to his wisdom and heard his heart for people he has himself cared for. We heard the same philosophy from a later presenter, Dr Victor Montori, Rewoldt Professor of Medicine at Mayo Clinic. A diabetes specialist with expertise in shared decision-making (SDM), Dr Montori is the author of the book *Why We Revolt: A Patient Revolution for Careful and Kind Care.*[7] He led by showing a slide with a quote from the Making Care Fit Manifesto, created by 25 people (including him) from different countries and disciplines who came together in 2021 and published the manifesto online in *BMJ Evidence-Based Medicine.*[8] It says, "Patients and clinicians must collaborate in designing care plans that maximally respond to each patient's unique situations and priorities while minimally disrupting their lives and loves." Perhaps the most important word in the quote is "respond." It indicates that the person has spoken (or been truly seen and heard) first. Shared decision-making may not ensure the person literally speaks first but it does ensure the person's voice is invited into the clinical space and honored. (For more about SDM in cancer care, the ASCO Education Book from this meeting is an excellent start.)[9]

A key point about SDM is that it is a method of care, not an add-on. Just as the VA sees Whole Health as an approach to care and not a program, SDM is a mindset shift. To shift said mindset and get to something new, we need to talk with people who know things we don't. In this book, we will show again and again that these are the patients themselves and their loved ones. They know important things we as the care team don't know. It is part of our job to learn those things.

The group of 25 people who created the Making Care Fit Manifesto had an enormous range of lived experience as patients, caregivers, clinicians, and researchers. The supplement to the Manifesto lists:

> Patients had lived experience with ENT cancer, type 1 diabetes, or genetic disorders. Caregivers had a relation to a patient as a mother, daughter,

or partner. Clinicians were general practitioner, public health physician, nurse, internist, physician, junior physician, case manager, pediatrician, diabetologist, or diabetologist for young adults. Researchers with a focus on organizational psychology, vulnerable patients, placebo/nocebo effects, uncertainty, shared decision-making, patient-clinician communication, value-based health care, argumentation, ethics, sociology, epidemiology, and/or treatment burden. Designers with a focus on service design, design methods, and/or support tools. Policy makers were medical director or quality improvement specialist. Our collaborators were an ENT surgeon, a critical care clinical pharmacist, a psychologist, and a psychiatrist.

We share this to keep you thinking of the broader team and of who you can partner with as you seek to provide whole person cancer care (more on care teams in Chapter 3). Cancer clinics and centers could set up a smaller team to advance SDM in their organization and practice. The team doesn't need to be as large and varied as the Manifesto collaborators. Key members from the oncology team partnering with patient councils or representatives is enough. One Integrative Oncology Leadership Collaborative (IOLC) member, the team at Penn Medicine's Ann B. Barshinger Cancer Institute, expanded to include colleagues from marketing and communications to help connect patients to the team's planned next step of promoting wellness in survivorship. This also ensured that resources created would be engaging and effectively communicate with a broad range of patients.

PEER GROUPS AND COMMUNITY

Study after study has shown that social support is central to healing, yet many end up dealing with their disease isolated and on their own.[10] Many of our hospitals have cancer support groups, both general and diagnosis specific. Patients can also access local and national advocacy organizations for support. Online groups have proliferated. The challenge in many of these groups is that they're often not specific or focused enough on the age and stage of a patient for them to get a personalized benefit. For Jenny Leyh, being a young, pregnant person with cancer felt very isolating. "I hated the look of pity I would get from people in the infusion room. I was the youngest one in there by a couple of decades. Finding the Young Survival Coalition (https://youngsurvival.org/) was a game changer for me as I was able to meet other young women with similar diagnoses, many of whom were also pregnant or breastfeeding at the time of diagnosis. That support and talking to others who simply 'get it' shifted my perspective and made me even more confident in my treatments."

Often age, type of cancer, stage, gender, sexual orientation, and race are characteristics that can be used to match patients with support and help them overcome challenges of noninclusion. We will discuss the major gaps in cancer care and outcomes due to racial disparities in later chapters, but we note here that addressing racial disparities needs an explicit focus by cancer care teams. Other patients can find support more easily, but if we can help them save time in doing so (and in getting the right kind of support), we will be providing better whole person cancer care.

Consider keeping a list of reputable organizations in this realm to which you can direct your patients. National organizations and chat rooms can gather larger numbers to help form more specific groups of those with rare conditions. Properly matched and managed cancer support groups give people a safe place to share and learn from each other and can be online or in person, opening options for participation. Membership in a support group can also help reduce feelings of loneliness and isolation and reduce stress. If your institution has such groups for patients with particular diagnoses and demographics, and has found them well-received, consider founding similar groups for caregivers and family members. For guidance and training in group visits, including those for persons with cancer, see the Integrated Center for Group Medical Visits (https://icgmv.org/).

Like support groups but more personalized, buddy programs are another idea that may be particularly helpful for unsupported patients. Also known as peer support or peer mentoring programs, such a program may already exist in your institution—one that pairs the person with cancer with a survivor of the same type of cancer. Again, matching the person with the patient's demographics is key. Trust is crucial, and it is important for the peer to be able to authoritatively communicate with, access, and influence the cancer care team regarding the patient's needs. If a patient sees that a peer support person can get things done, they may be more likely to communicate their needs.

Finally, a growing proactive movement by cancer care teams to help patients become more engaged and empowered is by providing health and wellbeing coaches. These coaches are specifically trained in assessing patient readiness for behavior change. They know how to use evidence-based approaches to move patients along the readiness trajectory from education to engagement to empowerment, using techniques such as SMART goals and motivational interviewing. Some members of teams, like social workers, may be trained already in these methods. For those not trained, numerous programs for training in health coaching are offered around the country. Not all of these are designed for use in medical settings. The National Board for Health and Wellness Coaching (https://nbhwc.org/) sets standards and evaluations for health coaches and administers a national board certification program. Very few of these training programs focus specifically on cancer coaching and advocacy.

Using professionals trained or training in these or similar methods already is a good place from which to build. Licensed social workers (LSW) have many of these skills, including cognitive behavioral therapy techniques and motivational interviewing to support behavioral change. Enhancing that training with information on key lifestyle behaviors that help with cancer management (as described in Chapter 4) and providing links to community resources is a great way to assure quality patient engagement. In addition, these supportive encounters can protect patients from inappropriate use of the numerous untrained individuals who offer to help coach cancer patients through diagnosis and treatment. The online advice from many of those individuals and sites can be dubious and even dangerous.

THERE'S NO SUBSTITUTE FOR EXPERIENCE

Years ago, Dr Jonas worked with a very prominent pain scientist on a large, rigorous, randomized, placebo-controlled study of acupuncture for arthritis pain. The study was positive—showing that acupuncture worked to produce clinically and statistically significant improvement in patients' pain more than a placebo. Still, the researcher was skeptical and did not recommend it for patients. Then, he got debilitating back pain himself. He tried multiple other treatments, but they had little effect. Finally, he agreed to see an acupuncturist and after several treatments was largely pain free and back to work. From then on, he was a promoter and user of acupuncture for pain. While no one would ever wish for an illness just for the experience, this situation shows that experience can be even more important than data for clarity and motivation—even for scientists.

There's no substitute for experience but experience. We end this chapter with the voices of 2 people living with cancer and very much in control of their own care. Their voices remind us of who engagement is all about—the patient.

Suzanne, a 53-year-old woman with stage IV HPV positive anal carcinoma following a delay in diagnosis, shares how she engages in her treatment on a clinical trial:

> My physicians are so compassionate and are always asking me, as the patient, how I want to proceed. I am asked if I want to dial back the dosage on the trial drug to ease up the side effects or forge forward. I am briefed on my lab results weekly, giving me confidence in my overall health. This communication style and deference to the patient and the patient's tolerance is truly meaningful and makes me feel in the driver's seat.

I realize doctors in the business of treating cancer patients sign up for a tough job. They have to set realistic expectations regarding treatment, side effects, and prognosis before they've really had a chance to get to know you. It appears to me it takes a few appointments to build rapport and trust.

I try to remember my medical team is overworked, because they are, and that schedules are stacked. While not often, sometimes I have had to assert myself to make people slow down and really listen to me. This was critical when hospitalized twice during chemotherapy and radiation, my initial treatment course.

In health care, patients are a number. Demand what you need. Get an advocate to help you. I am a very strong-willed person, with the benefit of a high degree of education, who is trained to get what she wants. Not often, but on occasion I have to dig in with vigor and still cannot get the institution of health care to operate with a modicum of common sense.

I try my best to stay authentic with my medical care team. They need to know where I am physically, emotionally, and spiritually. One of my trailblazing doctors said to me, "We can always get better." This is true. No matter what the health challenge is, we can always find a way to get better in some regard.

HELPING WITH ONLINE RESOURCES

Many people turn to the internet for information and to engage with their diagnosis, manage expectations (and anxiety), and gain support as well as knowledge of cutting-edge treatments, out-of-the box considerations and, unintentionally, poor information sources. Tina is a 58-year-old woman living with lung cancer. She shares her experience and tips for managing this area:

When I was first diagnosed with stage IV lung cancer, I was alone in a hospital room and immediately took to the internet. The research paper I found that discussed longevity said stage IV lung cancer patients have months, at best. My heart sank. But then I read a little closer and saw the paper was about 10 years old. I quickly told my friends and family if they searched the internet for my type of cancer, they'd—unnecessarily—start planning my memorial service. I am an experienced health reporter but quickly went down the wrong path as a new cancer patient.

To educate myself about cancer and to find support from other patients and experts, I rely heavily on the internet. But I try to use it judiciously. Indeed, after that first scare, I stopped Googling about longevity and instead went to work to find a good oncology team. That took a little internet searching to see where I could get care and to read patient reviews. I met with a few different doctors. Then all those questions I had for Google, I asked my new oncologist and her team.

I trust and like my oncology team, but I wanted more support and sources of information than they could provide. I again turned to the internet, looking for groups that might help. I stayed away from groups that were run by someone trying to sell me something or didn't have a professional staff. I found one that paired newly diagnosed lung cancer patients with patients who are now cancer-free. From the person I was paired with, I learned about a lung cancer organization, Lungevity.org, that supports patients and advocates for lung cancer research. It is very well organized, has a professional staff, a scientific board of directors, and other indicators that it's a legitimate organization.

It offers online exercise classes, support groups, art therapy, and more. They are run by professionals in their fields, which is particularly important for support groups.

I learned about another support and advocacy group that is specifically for people with my type of lung cancer. The group is called ALK Positive, after the type of genetic mutation we have. This group has also proved invaluable. It has a professional staff, a board of directors, and a very active Facebook page, where patients post questions and updates about how they are doing. I've learned a lot from other people's experiences and advice. But I need to be careful not to go down a rabbit hole of reading all the questions and comments. When I learn about specific medications or treatments that sound helpful for side effects I'm having, I talk to my oncologist about them.

These examples of empowered, activated patients highlight how patient engagement is so important in whole person cancer care. But these stories also illustrate how a combination of assistance from the care team, tenacity on the part of the patient and their loved ones, and a coordinated effort of all involved is crucial in the healing of any person at the center of a treatment plan.

SUMMARY POINTS

- The patient is the ultimate decision-maker in their care.
- Our cancer treatment system disempowers patients and so undercuts their decision-making.
- Care teams need to be sensitive and proactive in helping patients engage—by educating them about the importance of whole person healing and inviting them to get involved.
- Decision aids and shared decision-making allow people to engage in their own care.

- Properly matched peer support groups and buddy programs are powerful ways to get patients engaged and empowered.

- Social workers and oncology nurses are well positioned to empower patients, and with training and support can be at the center of patient trust-building for whole person care.

- Taking time to listen and learn from people's experience is the center of patient engagement.

CHAPTER THREE

THE CARE TEAM

If we think of a team as a group of 2 or more people who function interdependently to achieve a shared goal, the shared goal is an essential (and some might say most important) aspect of the team.

Although many face a cancer diagnosis alone, others create goals for treatment that include loved ones, such as, "I just want to make it to my granddaughter's graduation" or "My partner and I are going on vacation, then I'll start chemo." Truly honoring people's goals requires acknowledging their larger context and its interface with the cancer treatment. To provide whole person cancer care, teams must expand to include the full scope of the person's life, including their caregivers. This involves people who are not there to treat the tumor—those helping with stress, social support, nutrition, activity, and quality of life.

Care team membership for people with cancer and their proxies may be the next step toward whole person care. If we objectify the cancer and invite the whole person into care planning (making/taking action), we can partner to get somewhere better, sooner. If shared decision-making (SDM) means that the best practice in killing the cancer is not deemed best for or by the person, that changes how we move forward. It remains our job to educate people in the wily ways of cancer, to ensure they know what they are up against when they make decisions. In this chapter, we touch on some of the roles needed within whole person care and how they can be integrated into teams with shared goals.

THE LARGER TEAMS

Most oncologists in practice in the US today weren't trained in the era of team-based medicine. That will change over time, but not before we all live through the shortage of oncologists, advanced practice providers, nurses, social workers, and others. A shortage that is already severe and predicted to worsen in the near future. Nurse practitioners and physicians assistants (also called advanced practice providers or APPs) have emerged as key providers that contribute to increased productivity and quality improvement within teams, even as the complexity of care has continued to grow. Teams are learning to utilize all members at the top of their licenses (or job descriptions) and adding skills to provide better care. What if we also leveraged all team members to support patients in meaningful behavior change and wellbeing? This means working with staff at all points in the clinical workflow to create a shared mental model of whole person cancer care. On such a team, the front desk staff has influence equal to that of the medical assistants and the pharmacists, nurses and physicians, social workers and financial counselors, and so on, should we be lucky enough to have all positions filled.

What if the care team concept was grown to its full conclusion and included the person with cancer, along with significant friends and family members as well? And what if the care team saw its role as not just killing the cancer, but in helping the person become healthier during the process and on the other side?

Health behavior change is usually of interest to people with cancer. Yet, supporting such change within routine oncology is one of our least developed skill sets. This is no fault of our care teams—learning to provide this support hasn't been historically stressed in medical education. Even when it's offered as part of training, discussing changes in the compressed appointments of actual practice becomes unrealistic. We need a new paradigm for offering support for behavioral change—including support at the highest levels of the health care system. This can be achieved. If a large system like the VA can pivot to Whole Health to "equip and empower people to take charge of their health and wellbeing, and live their life to the fullest," then other systems can likely do so too. A big change from the status quo is never easy or comfortable, but it can be done. We discuss this in more detail in Chapter 15.

Oncology turns out to be a great place to make these changes. In oncology we enjoy at times relationships that develop over years, built with trust and, we hope, from treatment to survivorship. Our field is ripe for supporting people not just to treat their cancer but their wellbeing throughout the process and beyond. A clear example is that in survivorship, health coaching is associated with improved quality of life, mood, and physical activity.[1]

THE ROLE OF HEALTH COACHING

To meet people with cancer where they are when they bring up issues surrounding health behavior change, having a health coach (whether a person formally designated or by leveraging skills of a nurse or social worker) at the ready can help seize the moment. After the clinician suggests a way the patient can engage in "healing assignments" as discussed in Chapter 2, those trained in health coaching can pick up the thread and help make it real for the patient. If you don't have health coaching on the team yet, training a current team member or making a referral might be appropriate. Health coaches are different from health educators. They help patients set goals and remove the barriers to achieving those goals. They utilize skills such as motivational interviewing, active listening, and behavior change. The National Board for Health & Wellness Coaching (NBHWC) has established standards for health and wellness coaching programs, and graduates from these programs are eligible to sit for the national board certification exam. NBHWC has collaborated with the National Board of Medical Examiners (NBME) since 2016 to provide a board certification examination. According to the NBHWC, more than 350 organizations are hiring HWCs within the US and over 9,400 coaches hold the NBC-HWC credential.[2]

If your health system is interested in supporting behavior change efforts for the record number of people surviving cancer, gathering data to share on the use of health coaches could lead to support for the coaching initiatives you may propose. As an example, Thomas Jefferson University's Sidney Kimmel Cancer Center completed a feasibility study of health coaching in prostate cancer patients.[3] Over a 12-week, no-cost digital health coaching program, men with prostate cancer received at least 1 phone call and up to 4 "digital nudges" on topics ranging from fatigue, pain management, healthy eating, exercise, managing incontinence, sexual health, managing stress and anxiety, financial toxicity, goal setting during treatment, managing side effects, communicating with the health care team, and medication adherence. Of the men enrolled, 71% completed the 3-month program, indicating that coaching programs are feasible.

For more data points to share with leadership when suggesting the benefits of health coaching for patients, download the Compendium of Health and Wellness Coaching from the *American Journal of Lifestyle Medicine*. The compendium lists numerous peer-reviewed coaching-related articles and provides in-depth information about the nature, quality, and results from each article in a detailed spreadsheet provided as an electronic appendix.[4] It's a valuable source of supporting research to help you argue the case for health coaching as a core skill on your team.

The VA has published data on virtual wellbeing services as offered within a Whole Health System of Care. Although not oncology-specific, a multisite group of providers and veterans involved in tele-Whole Health (tele-WH) services agreed to semistructured interviews to determine the perceived impact of tele-WH on veterans. Within the group, over 40% of the veterans had experienced tele-WH coaching or tele-WH education; the remainder experienced other modalities, such as yoga and tai chi. The dominant themes from the data included increased use of WH-aligned services; deeper engagement with WH-aligned services; and improvements in social, psychological, and physical wellbeing from the services.[5]

Health and wellness coaching is valuable for cancer caregivers as well, an acknowledgement of caregivers as integral members of the care team. In a recent case study of an adult daughter caregiver for a parent with a neuroendocrine tumor (NET), the 44-year-old described herself as her mother's advocate for the first 5 years after diagnosis. She then became her mother's primary caregiver while deprioritizing her own health, and she was diagnosed with obesity and anxiety. She came to telephonic health coaching at the suggestion of a NET patient advocacy organization, after expressing concerns about medications prescribed to her by her primary care physician to address her health conditions. Because she was interested less in using drugs and more in behavioral approaches, she undertook a 10-session health coaching journey that led to an eventual 15-pound weight loss at 1 year, with improvements in blood pressure and cholesterol and improved wellbeing, among other positive outcomes. The NET advocacy organization paid for the first 8 sessions and the caregiver paid for the final 2 sessions, subsidized at $20 each. Although this study documents just one caregiver's journey to health, it provides an example of the potential benefit of health coaching for anyone on the care team, professional staff included.[6]

Workplace leadership may be interested to learn the benefits of health coaching as a tool for quality improvement and staff retention. Many who come to health care do it to support health and not just to fight disease. Offering health coach training to team members who may be good fits can help retain them. As noted above, social workers already have many of these skills and some systems have trained care navigators in some health coaching skills. If a covered benefit in your system, encouraging employees to experience coaching firsthand could enhance uptake in the clinic for patients. One of the most effective ways to get buy-in from team members is to give them support and experience in self-care and wellness approaches that you are seeking for patients.

TRAINING RESOURCES FOR HEALTH COACHING

Numerous programs that focus on health coaching in a clinical setting are offered. When selecting a program, always look for one approved by the National Board for Health and Wellness Coaching (NBHWC). This organization provides the nationally recognized board certification examination for health coaches.

The Center for Excellence in Primary Care at UCSF, cepc. ucsf.edu/health-coaching-0

Offers online and in-person training for health coaches.

The International Nurse Coach Association, inursecoach. com/courses/

Offers Integrative Nurse coaching programs and certification for registered nurses, nurse practitioners, and nurse coaches.

University of Minnesota Earl E. Bakken Center for Spirituality & Healing, www.csh.umn.edu

Offers an integrative health and wellbeing coaching program.

Vanderbilt Health Coaching Certification Program, vumc. org/health-coaching/health-coaching-program

Designed for licensed health care professionals.

Wellcoaches School of Coaching, wellcoachesschool.com

Offers "Certified Health and Wellness Coach" path for credentialed health professionals. Endorsed by the American College of Sports Medicine (ACSM) and the American College of Lifestyle Medicine (ACLM).

Duke Integrative Health Coach Professional Training Program, dhwprograms.dukehealth.org/health-wellbeing-coach-training/about-dhwct/

Offers online-only or combination of online curriculum with instructor-led training.

AWCIM Integrative Health and Wellness Coaching Program, integrativemedicine.arizona.edu/education/lifestyle/im_health_coaching.html

Offers two certification pathways: Integrative Health Coach and Integrative Wellness Coach

ACLM courses on health coaching for health care providers, www.lifestylemedicine.org

Online continuing medical education courses, such as Coaching Health Behavior Change.

DREAM TEAM

In daring to dream a bit about what a team could look like in whole person cancer care, a health coach would be a welcome addition, especially since other team members are often fully occupied with their functions. If time could be allocated and there is enthusiasm for whole person care, consider how those roles could be filled by people on your existing team to bolster their interests. For example, nurses might be interested in joining professional societies such as the American Holistic Nurses Association (https://www.ahna.org/Resources/Publications/PositionStatements). In our experience, nurses are some of the most powerful change agents on any team. Ensure room for their unique skills, compassion, and enthusiasm to reach more aspects of the whole people in your practice. Build on their strengths.

As you and your team learn what others are doing in oncology, try to maintain curiosity rather than cynicism. How could your team add a support position or re-envision the workflow for getting a patient to see a nutritionist? Where did other teams find the funding for their initiative? How did they get support from their leadership? How did they engage their functional stakeholders, such as nursing staff and people with cancer? The current system thrives on the paralysis of skeptics. We are well trained, but overworked on initiatives that may not serve patients leads to cynicism and wariness around new ideas. As you evaluate the dream teams of others, listen for the background discourse that must have occurred to make them a reality. Then pick one and help get it into a quality improvement process.

MENTAL HEALTH: DR P COMES ABOARD

At the VA hospital where Dr McManamon works, Dr P, a clinical psychologist, was detailed to the clinic, physically co-located on the hallway where routine oncology care occurs. By the first week, Dr P found his way to veterans and family members in the waiting and infusion rooms, asked how we (his new colleagues) were doing, and in general made his benevolent presence known. Tellingly, he suggested we introduce him to patients as "our clinic's behavioral health specialist" rather than by his signature-line credentials. Already, this additional layer of care has become a great support to patients both in behavior change (such as smoking cessation) and in riding the roller coaster that follows a cancer diagnosis. Licensed Social Workers can also serve effectively in this way.

Even before Dr P's arrival, the oncology clinic used a group chat for direct access to the Primary Care Mental Health Integration team of psychologists, located some floors away. Through a secure monitored chat function, any staff member can message directly to request a warm handoff to the mental health service when needed acutely—for example, for a veteran with suicidal ideation. Our mental health providers are adamant that front desk staff and medical assistants be included in this function, and they are. Weekly, across 6 fellows' and 3 attendings' clinics, the service is tapped at least once, giving real-time support to veterans and team members in need. With the arrival of Dr P, our mental health support for patients has become even more robust and accessible.

In a survey of 1,455 cancer centers in the US, 85% indicated they offer inpatient and/or outpatient mental health services, although without granularity as to whether services are co-located with the cancer treatment site.[7] This is a welcome trend. It's inspiring to consider how we can work together to harness Whole Health in oncology at the VA and whole person cancer care elsewhere.

Naturopathic Doctor: Dr N

An emerging addition to oncology teams that is being tried out in several oncology settings is the inclusion of Naturopathic Physicians with specialization in oncology, ND FABNO (FABNO stands for Fellow of the American Board of Naturopathic Oncology and ND for Naturopathic Doctor).

NATUROPATHIC FELLOWS

Designation as a Fellow of the American Board of Naturopathic Oncology (FABNO) requires meeting a strict set of criteria including:

- 2-year Council on Naturopathic Medical Education (CNME)-accredited residency focused on naturopathic oncology, as determined by the ABNO Board of Medical Examiners OR in practice for at least 5 years with 2,250 oncology patient contacts AND

- Submit cases for review by designated examiners AND

- 50 CMEs in oncology-related topics

All approved applicants must then pass a board certification exam.

The ABNO core curriculum emphasizes the following:

- The evaluation and management of patients with malignancies, with an understanding of established standards and a multidisciplinary approach.

- Clinical experience that is focused on integrative patient management, coordinating care with medical, radiation, and surgical oncology, as well as palliative care and other integrative disciplines.

- Develop expertise to evolve one's clinical practice in the context of a rapidly developing area of specialization and complex patient management.

- Develop the ability to evaluate and conduct research.

Sandy Colvard, ND, FABNO at University of California Irvine's Susan Samueli Integrative Health Institute, spoke to the IOLC about how she sees her role on the cancer care team as safely anchoring care for people with an interest in the naturopathic approach. Many of us had never heard of her type of credentials, but FABNOs like Dr Colvard are accustomed to our unfamiliarity. As team members with shared goals, they can fill a gap in our knowledge base, allowing another layer of support for people who inquire about using supplements and natural products. Without this level of support, when faced with such a patient inquiry, our teams typically try to do a quick cross-check on Aboutherbs.com or another website geared toward safety. Or they ask a pharmacist, the unsung heroes of patient safety, for their recommendations. A practice ND can provide the robust data and advice we don't have the time or ability to find ourselves.

The next level of whole person care could be for your team to hire a FABNO, if you can. With surveys showing more than 80% of people with cancer use some form of natural medicine, the potential for unsafe interactions—and for benefits—are well-documented.[8] The University of California, Irvine used this approach to bring more integrative care into a breast clinic. The shortage of FABNOs means that telehealth could be a good option for consults.

An alternative to working with a FABNO could be partnering with a nutritionist who has done additional training in functional medicine or lifestyle medicine, such as a member of Dieticians in Integrative and Functional Medicine (DIFM), a dietetic practice group of the Academy of Nutrition and Dietetics (AND), whose members get training on the use of whole foods and tailored supplements. A dietician on your team might already be a member of AND, the world's largest organization of nutrition and dietetics professionals. This allows eligibility for reasonably priced training webinars through DIFM.

BASIC TRAINING IN INTEGRATIVE ONCOLOGY

Integrative medicine and health—the merger of complementary approaches with conventional care—is, like supportive care, part of whole person cancer care. Learning about integrative oncology can help teams better see where this knowledge and skillset fit. Building a dream team begins in small steps, like finding who on your team may already share interests, or where continuing education requirements can dovetail with providing whole person cancer care. For those on the team looking for more intensive training in integrative medicine and health, the Academic Consortium for Integrative Medicine & Health keeps a listing of programs (https://imconsortium.org/training-jobs/fellowships/). As of 2020, the Academic Consortium Fellowship Review Committee has set and monitored the educational standards for integrative medicine fellowship programs. For physician readers looking for a dedicated fellowship track in integrative oncology, programs such as the University of Arizona offer options. In 2021, Dr McManamon participated in the NCI-funded Integrative Oncology Scholars Program at the University of Michigan, which offered 100 select-ees (physicians, nurses, PAs, social workers, pharmacists and psychologists) working in clinical oncology environments, a 1-year curriculum in the knowledge and skills necessary to provide safe and evidence-based integration of complementary therapies into conventional oncology care. Such programs further uptake of team-based, integrative medicine as part of whole person care.

CARE COORDINATORS AND SYSTEM NAVIGATORS: LIFELINES AND GLUE

In the increasingly complex world of health care, the roles of care coordinator and system navigator are indispensable and filled by people who become lifelines for those with cancer. They are the glue holding our broken system together. If your practice is an oncology medical home, you most certainly have team members in these roles and know how they fill gaps to keep patient care safe and as efficient as possible. This may span from arranging travel support to and from appointments, to providing culturally sensitive educational materials, running new patient orientation groups, and addressing people's fears and questions to the best of their abilities in real-time.

These jobs are some of the most challenging on the team because they require deep interface with the system and the patient, and creative thinking to provide workarounds when care is unduly com-promised. Ask a navigator or care coordinator what they did at work yesterday and you may gain a deeper level of appreciation. Some of the best insights on quality improvement come from navigators.

Like discharge planners in the inpatient setting, navigators and care coordinators in the outpatient setting know the system, with all its flaws. As mentioned, they are often the best people to start with when considering a new practice improvement initiative, because they can provide input on whether the issue you are hoping to solve is the most pressing for people, and where the system is breaking down. Navigators most commonly have degrees in nursing or social work. There are also navigators and community health workers who may not have advanced training in the medical setting but who are experts at moving patients through the medical system, connecting them with community resources; sometimes they are more representative of the communities and cultures of patients seeking care. Care coordinator duties may have some overlap with utilization management duties and more typically deal with administrative and coordination needs. There is no commonly accepted definition for this role, but a graphic representation can be helpful:

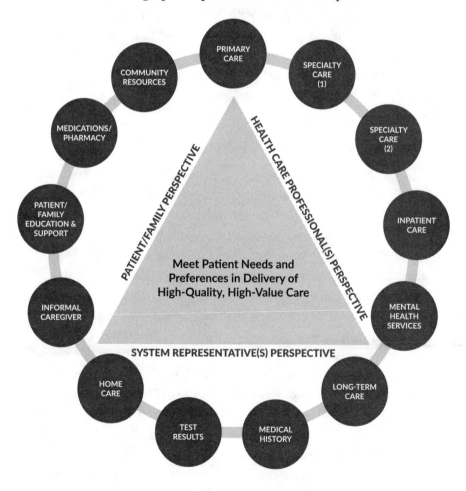

Figure 3.1 Care Coordination Ring
Adapted from Agency for Healthcare Research and Quality, Rockville, MD.
https://www.ahrq.gov/ncepcr/care/coordination/atlas/chapter2fig1txt.html

The ring shows the growing number of specialists involved in whole person care. Coordination of this care with the patient is becoming a major focus of quality improvement in health care delivery.

As can be seen from this figure, the complexity, and growing numbers of people on the cancer care team can be a navigation and coordination nightmare. Robustly trained and empowered navigators along with some of the practice redesign approaches described in Chapter 15, can engage and empower the team through shared goals and move the nightmare toward the dream. For staff members with interest in furthering integrative care navigation for patients, the Institute for Integrative Oncology Navigation at the Smith Center for Health & the Arts in Washington, DC offers formal training online (https://smithcenter.org/institute-for-integrative-oncology-navigation/).

THE ROLE OF PATIENT ADVOCATES

All of us on care teams may feel we are advocating for our patients all the time, yet the complexity of care means that we have blind spots. The medical system patient advocate, a clear-eyed presence employed by the larger system to represent the patient, can listen to the person with cancer describe events when something in their experience has gone awry. The patient advocate is tasked with trying to resolve the issue for the person. This balance of loyalties is not an easy task, as anyone in that role can tell you.

More simply, an advocate is someone in the corner of the person with cancer, usually someone who holds a dual role as a family member or friend and who speaks up on behalf of the person. Often these advocates are not familiar with the medical system; even if they are, they may have variable effectiveness with the larger team. Rarely, the advocate may be someone from outside the health system, hired by the person.

As care providers, we consider everyone on the team as a potential advocate for the patient. Even within the team, however, it's always a good idea to encourage a patient to consider who is their best advocate on the team and to add one if none exists, even if by assisting those who come with the patient into the role. Coming to your own aid is not something people should be expected to do, but many cancer survivors describe themselves in this role. When they do, it can mean that there wasn't a safe space for them to raise a red flag earlier in the care process. That matters. We can do something about it by encouraging people to see family members and others who often accompany them as advocates, as having the right to speak up. These advocates should be invited to the team and can be recruited to help the patient do their "healing work" between visits as described in Chapter 2.

A reframing of the role of the patient and using what matters to them as a guide for any advocate on the team can lessen the

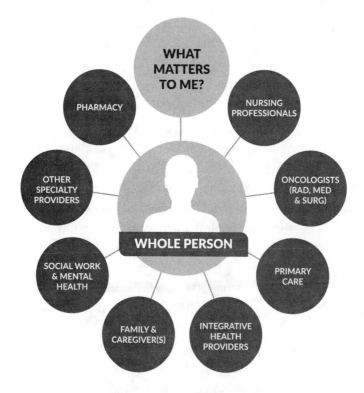

Figure 3.2 Treating the Whole Person with Team Care

What matters takes a central seat at the care planning table. The top circle becomes the central focus of team members trained as health navigators, coaches, or advocates. This role assures that team coordination does not all fall on the patient and is also not lost in the complexity of care.

coordination confusion and keep advocacy for what matters to the person from being lost in the process. Figure 3.2 shows a reorganization of the AHRQ Care Coordination Ring, with the patient as whole person in the center and the guidance of "what matters" taking a seat around the table (so to speak), weighted heavily in order to guide any team member or advocate, provider, or caregiver as treatment planning proceeds.

FORMER PATIENTS: THE WISDOM OF LIVED EXPERIENCE

Former patients can be outstanding team members, acting as patient advocates and peer mentors. The experience of a patient advocate who participated in the Integrative Oncology Leadership Collaborative (IOLC) is a great example. Yolanda "Yoli" Origel is founder and executive director of Cancer Kinship (https://www. cancerkinship.org/), an advocacy organization in Orange County, California that offers the Cancer Connections Peer Mentorship Program, among others. The organization's work grew out of Yolanda's personal experience following cancer diagnoses in her mother and sister and her own story of survival following BRCA1 positive breast cancer. Yolanda shares, "A year after treatment ended, I started mentoring patients at my breast surgeon's request. For every 10 people I mentored, 9 probably asked me, 'How can I do what you are doing? How can I help someone when I finish my treatment?'"

In an academic setting, Dr McManamon invited survivors from Walter Reed National Military Medical Center's John P. Murtha Cancer Center into a pilot to teach preclinical medical students about their experience since the time of diagnosis. The pilot additionally aimed to teach students how to use EHR and NCCN guidelines to create a survivorship care plan (SCP). The goal was to help students learn from people's mapped experience, drawn from the time of diagnosis to the present, and incorporate the 2 parts. After that, the oncologist, patient, and student met to finalize a whole person-informed SCP.

The results, presented at ASCO's 2017 Cancer Survivorship Symposium, showed that patients were willing participants and often asked for next step opportunities in teaching, having found additional meaning in their experience through this invited role.[9] As another example, Jan joined the Ovarian Cancer Research Alliance medical student training program (https://ocrahope. org/), where she taught medical students about patient needs for advocacy at several schools around the US.

Patients who show interest in helping others can at the very least be kept in mind as invited stakeholders when your clinic looks to start a new initiative in whole person care. As with any research or project involving patient care, we do best when we include the patient voice in the planning process.

THE LARGER TEAM: UNDER A BROAD TENT

Oncology pharmacists, nurses, radiation oncologists, surgical oncologists, interventional radiologists, art and music therapists, nutritionists, speech therapists, prehab/rehab specialists, exercise oncology professionals, pastoral counseling, other specialty providers, social workers, advanced practice providers, naturopaths, and primary care providers all have a role to play in whole person cancer treatment. The tent is broad and can't be too full if it aligns well with what matters to the person. Only your teams know what new role(s) would make the greatest difference for people where you work. Share your dreams with whoever is already in the tent as a first step. Integration with primary health care is essential. Chapter 15 and the Healing Works Foundation website give many examples of how cancer clinics and centers have used various team configurations and trainings to improve whole person care.

PRIMARY CARE: PARTNERSHIP

As the Institute of Medicine's 2005 call to action report on survivorship, *From Cancer Patient to Cancer Survivor: Lost in Translation,* approaches 20 years from its original publication, the ties between oncology and primary care teams remain little changed.[10]

Survivorship care plans haven't lived up to their full promise, through no fault of any party working within the system. To remedy this, models for shared but parallel care or for embedding a primary care physician and/or advanced practice providers (or 2) into long-term survivorship clinics are ongoing. The bottom line remains that as more people with cancer survive, we need to create lines of communication and education that don't rely on the patient as sole go-between in cases where they do transition back to primary care, as most survivors typically do.

When any large initiative is proposed in your cancer center, a good start is to integrate a representative primary care provider from bodies such as the American Association of Family Physicians (AAFP) or American College of Physicians (ACP). Notably, the Panel and Sub-committees for the NCCN Guideline 1.2022 on Survivorship included a handful of internists, some of whom were oncologists, and no family medicine providers. Within your own institution, inviting a primary care leader as a stakeholder can provide valuable insight as you create something that you hope will benefit those they lead and those under their care. From the authors' perspective as a family medicine physician and a hematologist-oncologist, we are working toward a shared goal: to make whole person cancer care routine and regular. The partnership reinforces what drew us to help others in the first place.

A FINAL WORD ON CARE TEAMS

Within any team, made up as it is of multilayered individuals, no one member can escape the relational complexity. Teams change—people leave, some get burnt out, priorities from leadership or system changes descend on the team, new workload, and finance issues surface. Team success or failure sometimes hinges on the smallest dynamic between even 2 of many members. It serves us to be very clear as to who is on the team and to invite members to play to their strengths. It serves us all to have leadership backing when there is a need to disinvite and assist anyone who can't function well on the team or who is impaired for any reason. In oncology, as in most fields, we have seen both. To help our patients we must first help ourselves. Please don't remain silent when there is a problem on your team.

SUMMARY POINTS

- Good cancer care is now done by teams, working in a coordinated role to benefit patients.

- The patient and their support persons are an integral part of the team.

- Whole person care requires some new or enhanced skills and staffing.

- Exploring new team members and different integration approaches may be helpful.

- Examples of new models are embedded behavioral and mental health, primary care, naturopathy, integrative health training, health coaching, patient advocates, group visit design and others.

- The wellbeing of the oncology team is what allows sustainability of good care.

CHAPTER FOUR

WELLNESS AND WELLBEING

While cancer and its management are complex, the core wellness factors that facilitate healing are conceptually simple. There are mostly a set of behaviors, that if made habitual, enhance our inherent healing capacity, improve our quality of life, prevent disease, and prolong survival. They are basic factors that an extensive body of solid research has shown improves the quality and quantity of life for anybody at any time, with or without any disease, and regardless of diagnosis. They are key to a flourishing life. And they also support health, healing, and wellbeing in people diagnosed with cancer. Most of them involve behavior and lifestyle.

These core wellness factors can also act as tools for empowering patients in their own care. Whole person care emphasizes their importance and educates and supports people to incorporate them throughout the cancer journey. Things that facilitate healing are also important for care teams and caregivers to know and utilize themselves. They help improve clinical wellbeing and blunt the forces of burnout.

In addition, the most direct and efficient way to move your team toward whole person care delivery is to apply these factors first with your staff, including clinicians—healing the healers. In Part Three of this book, we provide specific resources and tools for enhancing self-care and wellness. In this chapter, we describe the science that underlies those tools and justifies prioritizing them for everyone involved—patient, caregivers, and care team members alike.

As you read this chapter, think also about how these core wellness components present in your own life.

CORE WELLBEING FRAMEWORKS

There are many frameworks describing what humans need for flourishing. However, all of them are basically different ways of describing what we call the core wellness factors. Almost all modern frameworks have origins in Maslow's Hierarchy of Needs (see Chap-ter 1). Two of our favorites in the health arena are

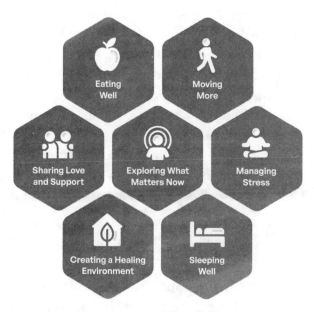

Figure 4.1 The Seven Healing Practices
Used with permission from CancerChoices (https://cancerchoices.org/healing/ 7-healing-practices/). A framework for enhancing health and wellbeing of people with cancer. Note that our "Core Wellness Factors" described in Chapter 4 are a modification of these and others.

those developed at the University of Minnesota Earl E. Bakken Center for Spirituality and Healing (https://www.takingcharge. csh.umn.edu/) and the VA's Whole Health model (www.va.gov/ WHOLEHEALTH). Neither model, however, was developed specifically for people with cancer. For that, we like the model used by the website CancerChoices (www.cancerchoices.org), a program of the nonprofit Commonweal. A 2021 quality assessment by NCI experts of online complementary and integrative medicine information resources ranked CancerChoices (at that time branded differently) at the top of 15 sites.[1]

Figure 4.1 is a graphic adaptation of the CancerChoices' Healing Practices framework and shows how the components are interconnected into a health-promoting, evidence-based whole.

THE CORE WELLNESS FACTORS

The core wellness factors apply, like Maslow's hierarchy of needs, to all human beings. For ease of implementation in routine care, we have simplified them further and integrated them into the 4 domains of the Personal Health Inventory (PHI), and the Healing-Oriented Practices and Environments, HOPE Note Toolkit described further below. While these components are the same for everyone, with or without cancer, specific areas may be more important for any individual, depending on their needs. They may be adjusted or modified, depending on the stage of cancer, status of treatment or survivorship, and readiness of any particular patient. Our simplified 7 core wellness factors are as follows:

1. **Learning:** Giving back to others or society by focusing on what truly matters. Detaching from nonmeaningful activities is part of that process.

2. **Loving:** Having deep and satisfying social relationships with family, loved ones, friends, neighbors, colleagues—anyone who's important to you. Quality, not quantity, is what matters.

3. **Relaxing:** Being able to relax deeply and remove yourself from the stresses, strains, and worries that are an inevitable

part of life. Activation of the relaxation response is a skill that can be taught and strengthened.

4. **Sleeping:** Deep and restful sleep, usually at least 7 to 8 hours a night.

5. **Eating:** A balanced, nutritionally dense, minimally processed, mostly plant-based diet, not too much and not too little, supplemented with extra nutrients and calories, as needed.

6. **Moving:** Movement routinely built into daily life through normal activities and exercise to maintain strength, flexibility, and good circulation.

7. **Being:** Immersing oneself into a physical environment that is restorative and helps the body heal and recover. For some, connecting with a higher power.

When people with cancer can incorporate at least some of these core wellness factors into their daily life, they build a supportive set of healing-oriented practices and environments around them. While improving even 1 factor (sleep, for example) can produce major benefits, optimizing as many factors as possible multiplies their effects substantially. Because many people with cancer have comorbidities such as heart disease or diabetes, and many now survive years after or with cancer, applying these factors can help improve overall health.

HEALING AND CURING

Eliminating the tumor is important in treating cancer—the focus is curing. Equally important is modifying the environment in which cancer grows—the focus is healing. Whole person care integrates curing and healing. Applying the core wellness factors can improve cancer care by reducing side effects, helping people get through the experience with less stress and a more optimistic outlook, and synergizing with other approaches that influence the hallmarks of cancer and the tumor microenvironment that we will discuss in Chapter 5.

The core wellness factors also help make the body less favorable to cancer and so reduce the risk of recurrence or a second cancer. In addition, they can help reduce cancer's long-term impacts and let the person return to a full life, sometimes even healthier than before the diagnosis. We recommend introducing the wellness factors early in the cancer journey as a tool for empowering patients in their own care.

When we present the wellness factors as part of cancer management, different patients pick up on different aspects and implement them at different paces. That's fine. Some will be drawn to one and struggle with others. Jenny dove into yoga and mindfulness. Jan emphasized the social and spiritual factors. Both used acupuncture. Some people won't be interested in any self-care approaches and may benefit from gentle nudges as their cancer journey and their readiness changes. Others will go overboard on factors such as diet and supplements and will need to discuss the evidence balancing related benefits and harms. Let's now look at each of these wellness factors and review some of the evidence for them in cancer care. In Chapter 12 we lay out tools and resources for implementing each of these factors in practice. In Chapter 13, we discuss the use of referrals and extended professional services to also enhance their use.

LEARNING: WHAT MATTERS

Although no one wellness component is more important than another, knowing what gives meaning to a person's life—what matters the most to them—is central to whole person care. Some consider it an existential or spiritual topic. It is, in many ways, the driver of life and action. This knowledge helps teams focus on how to personalize treatment and motivate engagement. For example, if what matters most to an older person with cancer is being present for their grandchildren now, their treatment might focus on quality of life and symptom control more than curative intent or longevity. If cancer comes to a younger person when they have small children or are pregnant, length of life takes priority. The life priorities that count most are where most patients will want to spend their time and energy.

Some people come to cancer already having a strong sense of what's most important to them. For them, that purpose doesn't change much over the years. But for most people, what brings the greatest meaning and joy evolves and shifts with age, especially if they continue to learn and grow.

Others may need encouragement and some direction to begin thinking through what matters and how they want that to influence their treatment. The process may take some time—few people think as deeply about these questions until cancer focuses their attention. A cancer diagnosis may offer an opportunity to focus on these discussions. Giving people the tools and time to step back and look more deeply at what matters becomes important.

Finding and expressing your deepest feelings isn't always easy, even for people who are normally articulate and open. Clinicians need excellent communication skills to initiate these conversations and make them meaningful. The 2017 ASCO consensus guideline on patient-clinician communication is a helpful starting point even for those who consider themselves good communicators.[2]

While the team oncologist may not be the one to have an extended "what matters" conversation with the person, they do need to support the process and encourage its use. This helps the team address all the core wellness factors. Consider how nurses, social workers, patient advocates, psychologists, and others with similar training and common tools may be equipped to have an open and meaningful conversation to inform the care plan.

When personal conversations aren't working, or the time to have them just isn't possible, some tools from the HOPE Note Toolkit can be helpful.

The HOPE Note Toolkit

The HOPE Note Toolkit is essentially a place to learn about and document the underlying determinants of a patient's health, including their values, priorities, and goals. The HOPE questions can help people express what matters to them, while also helping build trust within the therapeutic relationship and giving direction to the treatment. The questions help patients articulate their desires and priorities and what they want for their future after a cancer diagnosis.

The first HOPE questions are designed to learn what the patient finds meaningful, what motivates them, and what provides them with a sense of well-being. In other words: "What matters?" versus "What's the matter?" Some additional questions along the same lines might include: What are your plans and aspirations in life? What is your purpose? What brings you joy? The discussion is easier to have if the patient fills out the Personal Health Inventory (PHI) before the visit, providing an opening for the discussion. We mention these tools now and then and in Chapter 11 we give detailed examples about how these tools are used.

Exploring what matters evokes deep and sometimes personal questions, ones that perhaps the person with cancer hasn't yet given much thought to. They may not be answered immediately or completely when first asked—or ever—especially if a trusting relationship with your team hasn't yet been established. Timing on when to have that discussion is usually after the first or second visit once the tumor treatment plan has been created.

Dr Donald Abrams, Professor Emeritus at UCSF and author of the textbook *Integrative Oncology*, advocated asking 3 questions to open up a conversation about what is meaningful for a person with cancer—What brings you joy? What are your hopes? Where does your strength come from? And then pause to listen.[3]

Reflecting and Journaling

Besides a HOPE visit, just having a process to reflect privately on what matters helps clarify what is true for a person. Journaling is an excellent method for reflection, both for team members and patients. Also known as therapeutic writing or expressive writing, journaling encourages thought about values and priorities. A journal also provides an outlet for negative thoughts and difficult or uncomfortable emotions that the person may not want to share with others.

Journaling has proven benefits for managing stress and decreasing symptoms of depression and anxiety.[4] Journaling can also help decrease physical symptoms. A study of journaling for women with early-stage breast cancer showed that those who journaled their thoughts and feelings during treatment had fewer medical visits for cancer-related physical symptoms.[5] Another study looked at journaling for people with renal cell carcinoma. Those who journaled had fewer cancer-related symptoms and improved physical functioning.[6]

LOVING

The second wellness factor is in the broad category of love and belonging, something that matters to most people.

Social Support

Research has demonstrated the value of close ties and social support for cancer patients. The evidence is so strong that the SIO 2009 guidelines for complementary therapies gives social support a Grade 1A rating—the highest recommendation for evidence, safety, benefits, and being applicable to most patients.[7]

Social support helps people with cancer adjust to their disease and is crucial for helping them maintain a good quality of life throughout treatment and during recovery and survivorship. Social support comes in 3 basic flavors: emotional (feeling loved and having someone to trust), instrumental (someone to provide immediate help), and informational (receiving advice or information). The evidence for the value of social support in all 3 dimensions is broad across the cancer spectrum. The cancer care team can assess a person's social support level through the social and emotional questions of the HOPE Note Toolkit, which ask about support from family members and friends. If there is a need in this area, involvement of social workers, support groups, or a cancer buddy might help.

People with good social support networks are less likely to suffer from anxiety and depression, have fewer or more manageable side effects and physical symptoms, and may recover more quickly from surgery and the effects of chemotherapy. To cite one example out of many, a recent study looked at the importance of social support for optimism, resilience, and quality of life in cancer patients. Satisfaction with the sources and types of their social support from friends and family related positively to their quality of life, improved their general health, helped them cope with their disease, and reduced physical symptoms.[8]

Good social networks even impact death from cancer. In a meta-analysis of the associations of social networks with cancer mortality, having high levels of perceived social support, a larger social network, and being married were associated with significant decreases in the relative risk of death. High levels of social support reduced the relative risk for mortality by 25%; a larger social network by 20%; and being married by 12%. People who were never married had higher mortality rates than widowed and divorced or separated patients.[9] Clearly, social support is a key component of whole person cancer care. One of the mechanisms through which social support may work is through the mitigation of loneliness (an epidemic in modern society), which influences not only our social and emotional life, but the immune and inflammatory drivers of cancer.

Finding Support

When people with cancer don't have much support, the care team can help by putting them in touch with cancer buddies, support groups, social workers, psychologists, chaplains, and others. Given the known detrimental effects of lack of support and loneliness on outcomes, this is an essential part of whole person care; first ask about it and then bring in social workers, chaplains, and others to help early on. Many times, the kindnesses shown in cancer care visits goes a long way toward the relationship building that leads to mutual support. In this way, we serve and receive.

RELAXING

Decades ago, Dr Hans Selye described the core psychobiological response to threat and the damaging effect of repeated threats.[10] He and others have shown that repeated threats erode resilience and healing capacity and increase the chance of breakdown and further disease, including cancer.[11] Fear produces stress. A cancer diagnosis and its ongoing treatment and monitoring are practically synonymous with repeated threats and fear.

Fortunately, we have several ways to help mitigate stress, mostly involving the core wellness factors. Collectively, a variety of mind-body methods can blunt and mitigate the stress response directly, as shown by Dr Herbert Benson at Harvard. He coined the descriptive phrase "the relaxation response" and demonstrated practices that invoke relaxation counter the stress response and can modify genetic expression of cancer hallmarks, affecting metabolic and inflammatory pathways such as NF-κB, known to have a prominent role in inflammation, stress, trauma, and cancer.[12,13]

Stress, depression, anxiety, pain, and insomnia all respond well to a range of relaxation techniques, including mindfulness-based stress reduction, imagery, autogenic training, biofeedback, hypnosis, and meditation. The basic techniques can be self-taught with an app or online, or learned at free or low-cost classes through hospital systems and community centers.

The evidence for the value of a range of mindfulness and relaxation techniques on just about every aspect of cancer is extensive and strong.[14] Relaxation response methods are a core self-care wellness skill available to us all.

SLEEPING

Sleep is an essential part of health. It is when the body cleans itself of toxins, processes and integrates stress and trauma, and restores biological function. Its disruption, either in quality or quantity, increases risk for development and progression of cancer, and affects the major hallmarks of cancer, including immune function, metabolic and nutritional factors, and inflammation.[15] Poor sleep makes it more difficult to deal with the mental and emotional stresses of cancer and treatment. Even 1 night of inadequate sleep can impair immune function; prolonged periods of insufficient or poor-quality sleep are even more damaging.

Getting enough sleep is crucial for people with cancer. For optimal health and wellbeing, the American Academy of Sleep Medicine and the Sleep Research Society recommend that adults aged 18 to 60 years get around 7 hours of good-quality sleep every night. Surveillance statistics from the CDC tell us that 35% of Americans aren't getting the amount of sleep needed to protect their health. Sleep disorders are estimated to affect somewhere between 10 and 30% of all cancer-free people in the US. For people with cancer, the number is much higher: 59% of cancer patients experience disordered sleep.[16] On top of all this, cancer treatment frequently disrupts sleep.[17] Sleep disturbances can be very frustrating for people with cancer—at a time when good-quality sleep is important for rest and healing, they have trouble getting it. Untreated preexisting sleep issues such as restless legs syndrome, sleep apnea, and chronic insomnia, if still in place, may be worsened by cancer treatment.[18] A visit to the sleep lab may reveal treatable sleep issues unrelated to cancer, such as sleep apnea. Prechemotherapy and prescan medications, such as prednisone, can disrupt sleep for days. Long-term use of narcotics, alcohol, and sleep drugs disrupt the quality of sleep. For all these reasons, nondrug approaches for improving sleep in people with cancer are essential.

The whole person approach to better sleep is to try nondrug methods until something works. Start with the standard sleep hygiene advice recommended by the CDC, NIH, the Sleep Foundation (discussed later in this book in Chapter 12). People with cancer are already usually taking a number of drugs; nondrug approaches that avoid sedatives and sleeping pills such as iCBT are a safer approach.[19] People with cancer may not mention sleep problems to the care team. They may self-treat the problem with alcohol or use other drugs. They may feel little can be done for sleep, or they may be trying to tough it out—or maybe nobody has asked them about their sleep. Caregivers are also at risk for poor sleep. They too are kept up by worry over their loved ones and may also experience fragmented sleep from helping the person with cancer during the night. Their lack of sleep may impact both their ability to provide care and their moods, judgment, and health. Ask people about their sleep. While not written specifically for cancer patients, an overview of nonpharmacological approaches to sleep improvement in the journal *American Family Physician* provides excellent general guidance. It includes some of the core wellness factors described also in Chapter 12.[20]

Sexual Health, Urinary Symptoms, and Sleep

In the cancer clinic, a discussion about sleep often leads into one of sexual health concerns and, in some cases, concerns for urinary symptoms affecting sleep, most typically in men treated for prostate cancer. Appropriate referrals, such as to a sex therapist as when body image changes or medication side effects are affecting sexual enjoyment or to a pelvic floor therapist, when pelvic pain or urinary symptoms predominate, are important. People suffer when there are unmet needs in these areas, so asking with a plan in mind to help is important.

EATING

"Let food be thy medicine," said Hippocrates, and almost every prominent medical teacher since then has concurred. After smoking, poor diet is considered the most important risk factor for illness, including cancer. In fact, diet is estimated to be related to 30 to 40% of all cancers.[21] While the internet is full of claims for multiple dietary approaches for treating cancer, these remain mostly untested—and some may be dangerous.

Most people, including cancer patients, need to improve the basics of their nutrition. Fortunately, we know that a healthy diet is balanced, nutrient-dense, varied, and made up of minimally processed, mostly plant-based foods.[22] It can be supplemented with extra nutrients (protein, fats, vitamins, minerals) as needed; in some cases, extra calories may be needed as well. Portion sizes are designed to be satisfying—not too much and not too little. A healthy diet also takes personal preferences, cultural preferences, and traditions into account. Most of all, a healthy diet tastes good and provides enjoyment.

Within these parameters, no one dietary approach is ideal. However, a Mediterranean-like diet, which emphasizes all the basic elements, has the most evidence and is a recommended starting point. It's flexible, tasty, and has health effects well supported by good research.

The Mediterranean diet is unfortunately in sharp contrast to the way most Americans now eat. Recent research estimates that ultraprocessed foods, defined as foods that are industrially manufactured and ready-to-eat or heat, now make up 57% of the standard American diet. For all cancers, a 10% increase in the amount of ultraprocessed food in the diet is associated with a significant increase (greater than 10%) in cancer risk.[23] On top of this, poor and processed diet contribute to obesity, a major risk factor in itself for cancer and cancer mortality.[24]

At a minimum, cancer care teams can spend time educating patients about healthier dietary patterns and recommending basic shifts in eating. Referral to a nutritionist can occur anytime during care. For those who can afford it, multiple companies now supply healthy food kits, customized to a patient's needs, that can be cooked at home with minimal preparation.

Dietary Changes

The whole person approach to health emphasizes a healthy diet appropriate for the individual. The same is true when the individual has cancer. While there's no one nutrient, food, or even dietary approach that is anticancer, voluminous research shows that a diet low in saturated fat (especially from animal sources), low in sugar and refined carbohydrates, and rich in fruits and vegetables, whole grains, olive oil, and fish can help enhance the benefits of treatment and make the body's terrain less hospitable to cancer. Dietary changes can also make treatment easier and help reduce side effects.

Many people with cancer are very interested in dietary approaches that will help kill cancer cells and keep them from coming back. A good example of how well this can work is the story of Ken, a long-time colon cancer survivor. When Ken was unexpectedly diagnosed with stage III colon cancer in his 50s, his family swung into action to find him the best possible treatment. They researched oncologists who combined conventional and complementary treatments, a new and radical idea a few decades ago. They discovered Dr Keith Block and the Block Center for Integrative Cancer Treatment in Chicago. After surgery to remove the tumor, Ken traveled to the center to get conventional chemo-therapy every few weeks, accompanied by his wife. While they were there, they attended cooking classes and consulted with dietitians. As Dr Block says, "The cancer eats what you eat." In the classes they learned how to use whole, unprocessed, plant-based foods with known cancer-fighting potential to create healthy, delicious meals. They've used that knowledge ever since. Now in his late 70s, Ken is healthy, still active in his professional field, and remains cancer-free.

The philanthropist Michael Milken, a 30-year survivor of advanced prostate cancer, writes about his experience making major dietary changes as a component of his cancer treatment.[25] Given the emerging evidence for the influence of diet on the microbiome and the immune system described in Chapter 5, more attention to the food we eat not only for prevention, but also treatment is warranted.

MOVING

Movement routinely built into daily life helps maintain strength, flexibility, and good circulation. Our bodies are meant to move, and when they don't, health declines. The strong link between sedentary behavior (too much sitting) and cardiorespiratory risk has given rise to the saying, "sitting is the new smoking."[26]

The link between sedentary behavior and cancer risk is also strong, particularly for colorectal, endometrial, ovarian, and prostate cancer; it's a predictive factor in cancer mortality in women.[27] The evidence that regular physical activity helps prevent cancer is also abundant and strong, especially for colon, breast, endometrial, kidney, bladder, esophageal, and stomach cancers.[28] Walking for as little as 30 minutes a day lowers the risk of seven different types of cancer by 6 to 18%.[29] Movement is a core wellness factor for people with and without cancer. Because of this data, a growing number of cancer clinics are putting in routine services to help patients (and staff) get more movement.[30] Sharing information on movement as a cancer risk reduction strategy, and its positive effects on health and wellbeing can motivate patients who may not know the data.

Encouraging Movement

Whole person care encourages daily movement for everyone. The American College of Sports Medicine and the CDC recommendations for physical activity state:

- All healthy adults aged 18 to 65 years should participate in moderate-intensity aerobic physical activity for a minimum of 30 minutes on 5 days per week, or vigorous-intensity aerobic activity for a minimum of 20 minutes on 3 days per week.

- Every adult should perform activities that maintain or increase muscular strength and endurance for a minimum of 2 days per week.

These recommendations are based on the national physical activity guidelines from the Department of Health and Human Services.[31]

Physical activity during cancer treatment can be helpful for improving cancer-related health outcomes, including fatigue, quality of life, physical function, anxiety, and depression. It has also been shown to improve treatment-related symptoms in cancer survivors. This evidence is so strong that oncologists should consider an exercise prescription for all patients who aren't already active. The American College of Sports Medicine (ACSM) recommends asking people about their current physical activity at regular intervals; advising patients with cancer on their current and desired level of physical activity and conveying the message that moving matters; and referring patients to the appropriate exercise programs or health care professionals who can evaluate and help them exercise.[32] The team can ask about physical activity and point out its importance during visits.

A wide range of free and low-cost exercise options are readily available in most communities. Those who prefer or need a home-based, self-managed exercise program can easily find online options and videos, including many that are free or low-cost. Where available and needed, the care team can refer patients to health care provider supervised exercise programs, such as rehab gyms and physical therapy. Despite the ACSM recommendations dating back to 2019, payment, reimbursement, and availability remain barriers to supervised exercise. In our opinion, payment for services to help patients move should be part of standard cancer care coverage.

BEING

We mean by this term the physical environment, the space in which your body and mind exist. The hope is that this is an Optimal Healing Environment (OHE).[33] A full description of the OHE model is beyond the scope of this chapter, but we will point to a few tips and further resources that are most important for cancer care. These include regular exposure to nature and natural light, engagement in creative arts and music, and minimizing environmental toxins that may impair healing and promote cancer. For those with more interest, we recommend the book *Healing Spaces: The Science of Place and Well-Being,* by Dr Esther Sternberg, formerly at NIH and now at the University of Arizona.[34]

Regular Exposure to Nature

We evolved in nature, but modern life often removes us from it. Little surprise then that regular exposure to nature has beneficial effects on both mental and physical health, addressing several challenges faced by patients with cancer, including anxiety, depression, sleep, disconnection, stress, fatigue, and pain. Jan, who loved the ocean, would set up a wall hanging in her room during infusions or hospitalizations so that when she opened her eyes it looked like she was at the beach.[35] Studies show the influence of nature exposure on the immune system, including boosting the number of natural killer cells, a key part of cancer control for the body.[36] Even in the hospital, being in a room with a view and natural light facilitates wellbeing and accelerates recovery.[37] However, we don't know the optimal frequency and type of exposure for maximum effect. For now, patient choice and encouragement to do at least some exposure should be the guide.

Art, Beauty, and Creativity

Art, both viewing it and doing it, helps people access deeper learning and appreciation of life. Many cancer hospitals have artists in residence and music in residence programs to help patients facilitate recovery. Jan, who never thought she had any creative artistic skills, was visited by the artist in residence during one of her chemo infusion sessions. In that session, she discovered she had quite a knack for collage. This led her to join an art group and cultivate her newfound creativity. Artistic activity can improve patients' mental health, intuition, and insight.[38] Art and creative therapies are a standard part of the palliative care program at the NIH Clinical Center and are widely used at military and VA hospitals.

Music and Dance

Music may be a unique human experience. Babies exposed to music will spontaneously begin to move and dance. People, of course, vary in their response to music, but most enjoy it. A Cochrane review and meta-analysis of research on music interventions with adult cancer patients showed beneficial effects on anxiety, depression, hope, pain, fatigue, and quality of life. They also found that music may have a small positive effect on heart rate and blood pressure.[39] Music interventions in hospice and palliative care can help reduce anxiety, agitation, and pain for patients—as well as for family members and staff.[40] As with art, there is a difference between simply playing music and music therapy by a trained and licensed provider. Both can be beneficial and have their place. Few cancer centers have the latter.

Tobacco, Alcohol, Drugs and Other Environmental Toxins

There is no safe level of tobacco use. All people who use tobacco in any form should be encouraged to quit to protect every aspect of their health. To support them, offer enrollment in evidence-based smoking cessation programs. For people with cancer who smoke, quitting can reduce the risk of death. Extensive, mostly free resources are widely available to help people quit smoking. Hospital systems, cancer centers, local health departments, and community centers all offer quit-smoking programs. Apps, websites, and online programs abound. A good starting point for anyone wanting to quit is www.smokefree.gov.

Alcohol

Drinking alcohol increases the risk of cancer of the mouth, throat, esophagus, larynx, liver, and breast. The more you drink, the higher your risk. The risk of cancer is much higher for those who drink alcohol and use tobacco together.

People with cancer should avoid alcohol while undergoing chemotherapy treatment. Alcohol can interfere dangerously with some chemotherapy drugs, such as procarbazine (used in Hodgkin lymphoma and brain cancer). Liver inflammation from alcohol can block the effectiveness of some chemotherapy drugs or lead to heightened toxicities from chemotherapy or other medications such as painkillers. Alcohol can worsen nausea and vomiting side effects, interfere with sleep, and increase the risk of depression. According to the WHO, no amount of alcohol is safe for our health.[41]

Cannabis and Psychedelics

Cannabis and psychedelic drugs are not, technically speaking, toxins. But that depends on route and dose. These substances are active areas of research, mainly for their psychological and mental health potential. A full discussion of these is beyond the scope of this chapter but we will discuss the ones most used by patients. Marijuana and cannabis products such as hemp oil, THC, and

CBD have all been studied to manage cancer symptoms and the side effects of cancer treatment. They can help, especially with nausea and vomiting from chemotherapy drugs,[42] but the decision to use them is individual and may depend on state and local laws. People with cancer may be using these products without telling the care team—or they may ask the care team if they should use them. Be prepared with accurate information and nonjudgmental responses. IOLC members created a downloadable pocket guide on cannabis and cancer; it is available on the Healing Works Foundation and this book website. Jenny found cannabis very helpful for her nausea, anxiety, and sleep. Jan never used them and did not want to.

Environmental Toxins

There are many environmental toxins in our air, water, and food supply. Certain racial groups and those in poverty are often exposed at higher levels than the general population and for these groups they are a social determinant of health. To a degree some exposure is unavoidable, but exposure can be limited in some ways.

People with cancer often wonder if toxic exposure caused their disease. The NIH's 12th Report on Carcinogens lists 54 compounds as known human carcinogens.[43] The highest exposures occur in certain occupational settings, such as agriculture, but there are environmental exposures as well. If people with cancer bring up this concern, listen to understand what they may be asking. They are likely concerned for others they care about with the same exposure history or that they cannot be well if the exposure is ongoing. Radon, for example, is a natural radioactive gas found in many homes. A good source of information on the impact of the environment, including toxins can be found on the CancerChoices website (https://cancer-choices.org/healing-practice/creating-a-healing-environment/making-changes-in-your-environment/).

HOW TO SHIFT TOWARD WELLBEING: FOCUS ON THE TEAM

A shift from a sole focus on a *pathogenic* (disease treatment) mindset to include a *salutogenic* (healing and wellbeing) mindset and model may seem like a daunting task. We don't minimize the challenges this presents to the average oncology team. There *are* major system forces moving the other way. If you make changes, you will be stretched, swimming upstream, at least for a while. It helps, however, if you can build a boat and get as many of your colleagues in it, all rowing in the same direction. Both the evidence and rewards for making the shift are compelling. In Chapter 15, we describe several methods for and examples of systems that are now rowing toward whole person care.

SUMMARY POINTS

- Health and wellbeing are supported by a core set of health, healing, and wellness factors needed by all people, including people with cancer and those who care for them.

- These factors include learning what matters, love and social support, relaxation and sleep, healthy food and drink, moving more, and being in a healthy environment.

- These core wellness factors have extensive research to support their implementation in cancer care.

- People implementing 1 or more of these factors can improve multiple aspects of wellbeing.

- These factors are important in preventing cancer, while treating it, and after it is gone.

CHAPTER FIVE

HALLMARKS OF CANCER AND THE TUMOR ENVIRONMENT

Killing cancer, and killing it early, are key to both peace of mind and survival. However, killing cancer isn't the whole story. What surrounds the cancer—the tumor microenvironment—is also key to optimal treatment and survival. The tumor microenvironment is connected to the macroenvironment of the whole person, including the immune and metabolic consequences of their genetics and behavior. The micro and macroenvironments in which the cancer cell develops have as much to do with cancer regression as the killing of the cancer cell itself. Collectively, these environments are the scientific reason we need whole person care in oncology.

There's no better illustration of this than exploring how our immune system interacts with cancer cells. If the cancer cell didn't escape detection and destruction by our own immune system, it would never spread and be dangerous. The advent of "immuno-oncology" allows new approaches that manipulate this interaction. We now have novel drugs that allow the immune system to kill the cancer cell, and an expanded understanding of how lifestyle and wellness approaches facilitate this same immune modulation. We now have drug treatments that alter the metabolism of cancer cells, including inflammation and the nutritional environment of the cancer. Precision oncology, based on molecular profiling of tumors to identify targets for treatment, is mainstream. In addition, research shows that nutrition, behavior, lifestyle, and mind-body approaches can be used along with precision oncology treatments to produce or enhance those same molecular mechanisms, often in safe and synergistic ways.

In this chapter, we do a high-level review of that research and show how it provides the scientific basis for whole person care. We will first review 3 areas that influence the tumor microenvironment and are what are called the biological "hallmarks" of cancer. We will then illustrate how whole person cancer care influences the macroenvironment to affect those same hallmarks. Readers will then be more equipped to use the resources and tools of whole person care provided in Part Three of the book.

THE CELL GONE ROGUE

As the science of anatomy and physiology evolved, it gradually became clear what cancer is. Cells in specific tissues gone rogue, multiplying rapidly, breaking free of the normal mechanisms of control.

Cancer's growth rate is so astonishing that it far surpasses that of any normal tissues. So, removing the mass and slowing the growth of those cells became the goal and standard of all cancer therapy. This made (and still makes) complete sense. Regulatory requirements and investments backed this goal, developing the engine of research that creates new chemotherapies and the more targeted drugs we have today. The discovery of aberrations in gene expression added another dimension to our understanding of cancer biology—and new therapies have followed. This history and more are described in Siddhartha Mukherjee's Pulitzer Prize-winning book, *The Emperor of All Maladies*.[1]

There was only one problem with these approaches. They didn't work very well to keep most people alive. They worked well—even dramatically—in certain blood cancers (especially in children), and in lymphoma, testicular cancer, and a few other cancers, allowing people with those cancers to live on for decades. These were true breakthroughs. However, for most cancers, even when the entire tumor could be removed surgically or chemically and early on, the cancer often came back, usually with resistance to further treatments. For most people, complete or partial response (regression in tumor size) or progression-free survival (living for a time without tumor growth) doesn't mean prevention of recurrence or even a meaningful impact on long-term survival. In other words, these treatments often have little effect on overall survival and lifespan. In addition, therapies that are toxic to cancer cells are usually toxic to normal cells as well, producing side effects and reducing quality of life.

Today, we can know more about the biology of an individual's cancer than ever before. Sometimes this information helps decide the treatment—and sometimes it's just confusing. In Jan's second breast cancer, a genomic test helped determine a "recurrence score" and predicted that chemotherapy would increase her 5-year survival chances from breast cancer by 7%. A very low recurrence score would have suggested no benefit from chemotherapy, clearly something good to know when deciding on the best treatment.

As additional markers became available for Jan, a comprehensive genomic and proteomic analysis showed a dozen aberrations that were possibly driving her cancers, but hardly any had established drug treatments. Finding the BARD-1 gene mutation, for example, linked to an increased risk of breast but unknown risk in ovarian cancer, led her daughters and sisters to testing.[2] This led one of them to have her fallopian tubes removed and the other did not. Jan herself could take no action based on that discovery.

FROM THE TUMOR TO THE TUMOR MICROENVIRONMENT

From the earliest days of cancer research, investigators observed that the disease didn't always progress and wasn't always fatal. Even when family members inherit the same genetic mutations and are exposed to the same environments, some people never develop cancer. Others do, but their body controls or slows the growth, possibly even reversing it. While the cancer-killing paradigm grew and expanded, these scientific observations showed that killing the cancer was not the whole story.

It's now well established that the body is in a dance with cancer as it develops, progresses, and regresses. Multiple biological processes—the tumor microenvironment, or TME—surround the tumor and are part of that dance. We will review 3 key examples of that biology that help us understand the tumor microenvironment and its link to whole person care. These are immune-tumor interactions, metabolism and nutrition, and inflammation.

The Immune System

Early observations of immune-tumor interactions began with Dr William Coley, a Harvard physician in the 1880s who noticed that some patients who developed severe infections of the skin would have regressions of their advanced cancers. He tried to induce such infections in patients with cancer using injections of a bacterial mix that came to be known as Coley's toxins. He saw an increased number of them survive; some were even cured. Some of the infections he induced were quite severe, however, and patients did not always survive the treatment. The approach was used widely around the turn of the last century but fell out of favor as drug treatments and surgery advanced. Coley did, however, inspire further investigation into the role of the immune system in cancer management.[3]

Another early milestone in the role of infection and immunity was the discovery in the 1950s by Dr Denis Burkitt, who found that a type of lymphoma was caused by infection with the Epstein-Barr virus (EBV), further implicating the immune system.[4] This discovery had wide-reaching impact on many aspects of cancer research. Despite all the research in cancer immunology, no vaccine has yet been developed for EBV-associated cancers such as Burkitt's lymphoma and nasopharyngeal carcinoma. We still rely on intensive chemotherapy and/or radiation treatments.

Today we have a highly successful vaccine that targets human papillomavirus (HPV), the cause of cervical and some other cancers, including oropharyngeal cancer. Approved in 2006, this remains the only widely effective vaccine we have for cancer. We hold out hope for others, but the complexity of the TME implies that vaccines can be only part of the mix in whole person cancer care. After her first breast cancer, Jan received an experimental vaccine that seemed to prevent a recurrence or new cancer for years. On the other hand, after her ovarian cancer, she enrolled in a vaccine study that didn't prevent recurrence.

Fast forward over many researchers and decades to the 1990s, when Dr James Allison discovered specialized receptors known as checkpoints on some cancer and immune cells. The checkpoint receptors put the brakes on the immune system's ability to detect and target cancer cells. Checkpoint inhibitor drugs soon followed, which took the brakes off and let the immune system recognize the cancer cells. Dr Allison won the Nobel Prize in Physiology and Medicine in 2018 for his work. Immune checkpoint drugs are now widely used for a range of tumors. The results are sometimes dramatically successful, as with melanoma. But for many other types of cancer, they don't work very well. A major study on the heterogeneity (genetic variation) of ovarian tumors, even in the same person, illustrates the complexity and difficulty of a single treatment for cancer. The study showed that ". . . even personalized approaches may be ineffective against widespread and heterogenous disease within patients."[5]

Many other immune manipulation approaches have evolved along with checkpoint inhibitor drugs. These include CAR-T therapy, where a patient's T cells are modified in the laboratory to kill cancer, along with new vaccines, modifications of Coley's toxins that are less toxic, and other approaches that train the immune system to find and kill cancer. These treatments can produce effects in some patients, but many patients do not benefit.[6] However, immune manipulation is now firmly established as an important approach in cancer prevention and treatment.

Nutrition and Metabolism

Like all cells, cancer needs to have oxygen, nutrients, and blood flow to grow. Often, cancers hijack nutrients needed by other cells in the body. This knowledge has generated extensive research on the metabolism of cancer and has led many naturopathic and integrative physicians to recommend supplementing oxygen and reducing sugar in the diet. These approaches are unproven. The body carefully regulates both oxygen and blood sugar levels, almost independent of intake, so external manipulation likely has minimal effect on most cancers. Brain cancer may be an exception, further discussed below, especially when under radiation treatment.[7]

There is evidence that reducing nutrients to the cancer may help. As cancers grow beyond the microscopic level, they must also grow blood vessels to bring in nutrients and feed their ravenous appetites. Starting in the 1970s, the late Harvard researcher Dr Judah Folkman showed that if this process, called angiogenesis, is inhibited early on, it could interfere with cancer growth. Later specific factors that drive blood vessel growth, such as vascular endothelial growth factor (VEGF), were discovered. Building on this work, Dr Napoleone Ferrara developed the antiVEGF monoclonal antibody bevacizumab (Avastin®), approved in 2004. This drug is now used in combination with standard chemotherapy drugs to inhibit angiogenesis for many cancers. Results are variable because many other factors also promote angiogenesis, such as copper levels.

Inflammation

Normal inflammation is an acute healthy response to injury, infection, or tissue damage, designed to defend and repair normal tissues. Inflammation rises rapidly (and sometimes intensely) and then subsides as the threat is resolved. Systemic chronic inflammation (SCI) arises when the body is subject to repeated damage from the environment or from lifestyle factors such as obesity, smoking, or stress. SCI sets up an environment around cancer cells that drives cancer growth, spread, and invasion into other tissues, while blocking immune system surveillance.[8] SCI increases cancer risk and contributes to dysfunction and development of many other chronic diseases beyond cancer, such as diabetes, heart disease, and neurodegenerative diseases.[9]

Treatments targeting SCI are now a major area of research and expenditure for cancer and chronic disease. Because much of SCI originates largely in basic lifestyle and wellness factors, improving them is a safe and effective way to reduce inflammation overall. The low-hanging fruit in whole person cancer care is that almost all patients can implement healthy lifestyle changes that modulate SCI. Many patients choose to do so on their own; others can benefit from behavioral change assistance and encouragement from a health coach or behavioral therapist.

HALLMARKS OF CANCER: FROM THE TUMOR MICROENVIRONMENT TO THE WHOLE PERSON

The tremendous growth and knowledge about the TME over the last several decades opened a new way of thinking about cancer, its development, and management. We can summarize our current understanding by looking at 10 hallmarks of cancer, a concept initially proposed in 2000 by Dr Douglas Hanahan and Dr Robert Weinberg and updated regularly since then, most recently in 2022.[10]

The latest iteration of the 10 hallmarks of cancer is summarized in the call-out box.

Research is now showing that the microbiome may be an additional hallmark. Our body is colonized by a vast array of microorganisms—nearly 40 trillion cells—that live in and on us. As discussed below, researchers have found that some of these microorganisms can influence protective or deleterious effects on cancer development, progression, and response to therapy.

The hallmarks and enabling characteristics connect the biology of the TME to the tumor macroenvironment and the surrounding aspects of the person's mind, body, and behaviors; such as influencing the immune-cancer interaction though stress reductions or

THE BIOLOGICAL HALLMARKS OF CANCER

1. Self-sufficiency in growth signals. While normal cells depend on external growth signals for proliferation, cancer cells can generate most of the growth signals by themselves, greatly reducing or eliminating their dependence on external stimuli.

2. Insensitivity to growth suppressive signals. Cancer cells evade antiproliferative signals by subverting the mechanisms that control cell cycle progression.

3. Ability to evade programmed cell death. Cancer cells become immortal; apoptosis (normal cell death) no longer occurs.

4. Enabling replicative immortality. Unlike normal cells, cancer cells have an unlimited proliferative potential.

5. Sustained angiogenesis. The growth of cancer cells is fueled by growing new blood vessels that feed them.

6. Tissue invasion and metastasis. Metastasis is the cause of most cancer deaths. The ability to invade, settle in, and grow in distant tissues is therefore one of the main—and most feared—features of cancer.

7. Reprogramming energy metabolism. While normal cells use oxygen to process glucose and produce energy, malignant cells can switch to aerobic glycolysis even in the presence of oxygen (what is known as the Warburg effect).

8. Evading immune destruction. Normal cells that become defective are removed by the immune system. Cancer cells can evade detection and destruction by the immune system.

9. Phenotypic plasticity and disrupted differentiation. Increasing evidence indicates that malignant cells evade differentiation and unlock what is known as phenotypic plasticity to continue to grow.

10. Nonmutational epigenetic reprogramming. Cancer cells can reprogram a large number or gene-regulation networks to alter gene expression and favor the acquisition of hallmark capabilities.

Note: Adapted from Licciulli, S. New Dimensions in Cancer Biology: Updated Hallmarks of Cancer. Published in *Cancer Research Catalyst: The Official Blog of the American Association for Cancer Research*, January 21, 2022.

dietary changes that change the microbiome. This gives us a biological basis not only for new drugs and targeted therapies, but also helps us form an understanding and approach to whole person care.

CANCER HALLMARKS AND WHOLE PERSON CARE

Let's take the 3 areas of the TME just discussed and examine how they're connected to the hallmarks and the macroenvironment and how those are, in turn, influenced by whole person care. Figure 5.1 shows those areas surrounding the impact they have on the 10 hallmarks.

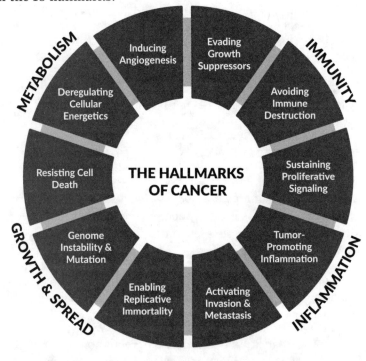

Figure 5.1 The Hallmarks of Cancer

The 10 boxes list the currently accepted hallmarks of cancer biology. Around those boxes are 4 physiological areas that influence those hallmarks and the behavior of cancer. In the chapter we describe how these areas are influenced by a person's behavior and the macroenvironment, making them levers for cancer prevention and treatment using whole person care.

(Adapted from Hanahan D. Hallmarks of cancer: New dimensions. Cancer Discov. 2022;12(1):31-46. doi:10.1158/2159-8290.CD-21-1059.)

Immunity

We've described the importance of optimal immune function in the control of cancer and the growing use of vaccines, cell modulation such as CAR-T, and drugs inhibiting immune checkpoints. We now know that many of the wellness factors described in Chapter 4, and resources to affect them described in Chapter 12, also influence the immune system and its function. Sleep is a good example. Disruptions to sleep and circadian rhythms alter immune function and increase the chances for immune escape, as when the immune system stops recognizing and eliminating mutated cells.[11] Patients with sleep disturbance do worse during treatment of cancer and have a poorer prognosis.[12] Those in jobs that regularly disrupt the circadian rhythm, such as shift workers, are at higher risk for developing cancer.[13] In addition, quality sleep improves quality of life and wellbeing—another reason it's a part of the core wellness factors of whole person care.[14]

Surgery can disrupt immune function and increase the chances of cancer cell spreading through mechanisms of postoperative inflammation, immune suppression and, at times, direct seeding of tissues.[15] While surgery is an effective treatment for many cancers, it's important that optimal immune function be supported and maintained before and after it by optimizing the core health and wellness factors.

Nutrition also influences the immune-cancer interaction. In addition to macronutrients such as high-quality carbohydrates, proteins, and fats—essential in managing cancer, especially in advanced stages—micronutrients such as vitamin D are also important. Vitamin D deficiency is common in cancer patients and can lead to immune dysfunction. While high doses of vitamin D supplements have not been shown to treat cancer, adequate levels of vitamin D are essential for optimal immune (and many other) functions.[16]

Stress Reduction

Stress and the mitigation of fear should be a commonsense part of all whole person cancer care, regardless of whether it has a measurable effect on the cancer or TME. While stress has not been shown to influence cancer progression,[17] the biology of stress and fear, the social environment in which people live, and the team's communication skills are important for wellbeing.[18] Recent research has shown that the brain-stress-hormone-gut connection and immunity are intricately linked, indicating that how we manage stress can influence the TME. Helping people with cancer learn to manage stress benefits their wellbeing. Conversely, patients with high stress levels or harmful coping methods usually don't do as well.[19]

Research on the placebo effect has demonstrated that belief, therapeutic ritual, and conditioning can result in important psychological and biological responses. As a good example, research has shown that pairing an immunosuppressive drug (for example, chemotherapy) with a benign conditioned stimulus (such as a sweet drink) can produce ongoing immune suppression when the conditioned stimulus (the drink) alone is given—even when the drug is stopped.[20]

Patients are already primed to react with fear when they hear the very word "cancer." If an authority figure such as a surgeon or oncologist delivers bad news without also providing an opening for hope, this only reinforces the negative expectation. The bad diagnosis can turn into the equivalent of a hypnotic induction, or what some cultures call a curse, with all the accompanying negative effects.[21]

Clearly, we need to be thoughtful and systematic in how we help patients manage stress and distress in all phases of cancer care. In addition, we can learn how to minimize the negative (nocebo) and enhance the positive (placebo) aspects of care. In doing so, we can manage both the psychological and possible biological impact of our communication and rituals. Better training in ways to deliver accurate information in an empathetic and healing way can be a key focus of any practice or program improvement in whole person care. Associate Professor Alia Crum, PhD and her team at Stanford Mind and Body Lab have developed and are testing a physician mindset training program to help clinicians avoid creating a nocebo effect through the way they label and communicate with patients (https://mbl.stanford.edu/resources/intervention-materials).

Nutrition and Metabolism

Nutrition and metabolism comprise another area where the TME is connected to the tumor macroenvironment and whole person care. We know that nutrition is important for the development, prevention, and progression of cancer. In addition to smoking and alcohol, the food we put in our mouths is another major contributor to cancer.[22] But can changing the diet change the trajectory of cancer, or even make it regress? Many alternative practitioners and websites claim it can—and many people with cancer are eager to believe them.

We've known for decades that unproven theories, such as Gerson Therapy based on one doctor's belief that nutritional deficiencies cause cancer, do not cure cancer. No radical diets have been proven to cure cancer. However, a connection of diet to cancer through the TME may be occurring through the diet's effect on the gut and the microbiome, the community of microbes in the gut.[23] Recent research has demonstrated that the composition of bacteria in the gut microbiome has a close connection to the immune system, and cancer development and its regression. One example is a rigorous study published in *Science,* which demonstrated that by using diet and fecal microbiota transplant to change the gut microbiome of patients who aren't responsive to immune therapies, some can be made responsive.[24] In addition, dietary changes that emphasize a diversity of plant foods and fiber can alter the microbiome in a direction less favorable to cancer spread.[25] The timing of antibiotic administration may also be important. Antibiotics disrupt a healthy microbiome and, if poorly timed, can interfere with the effectiveness of immune checkpoint inhibitors.[26] A healthy gut microbiome doesn't seem to depend on any one bacterium; rather, a diversity and balance of many organisms may be key. Cancer itself may disrupt that balance, providing a feedback loop that suppresses gut function, impairs immunity, and accelerates the cancer.[27]

Another popular dietary approach is the ketogenic diet, a high-fat diet that removes almost all carbohydrates (especially sugars). The diet puts the body into ketosis, which is claimed to enhance responsiveness to treatments in certain types of cancer. So far most of this research has been done on brain cancer. Since the brain requires glucose to function, brain cancers may be more sensitive to carbohydrate restriction than other cancers. Adhering to rigid ketogenic regimens, however, is difficult for most people. Time and further research will tell whether this is an effective addition to cancer care.

Fortunately, there's good evidence that one type of eating improves health largely across the board. For most people, including most cancer patients, the best recommendation is to start with a Mediterranean-style plant-based diet that's high in fiber and low in animal foods and sugar. The benefits may come not only from its nutritional superiority and high nutrient-to-calorie ratio, but its impact on the next cancer hallmark in the TME to whole person link: Inflammation.

Inflammation

We hear a lot about silent killers in medicine: environmental toxins, hypertension, diabetes, stress, and others. At the center of these killers—and probably of most chronic disease—is SCI. Inflammation, so helpful during acute injury, can be injurious if it is sustained, as when the body is not allowed to properly recover in between stressors. That recovery, in fact, is what keeps us metabolically, psychologically, and possibly even spiritually healthy. The biological term for this is hormesis (derived from the Greek, meaning "to excite"), or the stress adaptation response (SAR).[28] The SAR is the basis for maintaining fitness, resilience, and health. It occurs when any kind of mild stress or trauma, such as exercise, fasting, psychological challenge, or strong emotion, happens at a low dose or for short duration and is then removed. This allows the body to build its defenses and activate its repair, resistance, and recovery processes.

Hormesis is biologically and evolutionarily preserved across all living organisms, indicating its fundamental importance to survival. Extensive research now documents that many lifestyle and behavioral factors likely produce their benefit by reducing

SCI through hormesis.[29] The most comprehensive summary of this research, as well as its connection to behavior and lifestyle, was published in the journal *Nature* by David Furman, PhD and colleagues in 2019. This article summarized hundreds of studies showing that lifestyle and environmental factors influence SCI and these then drive many chronic diseases, including cancer.[30] Since then, other research and summaries have supported this understanding. Whole person cancer care programs that emphasis fundamental wellness factors support the hormesis process and reduce SCI.

FROM HALLMARKS TO HOLISM

As a practitioner or a patient, you're usually not long in the world of cancer before you run across recommendations for supplements and repurposed or off-label drugs (OLDs). OLDs are drugs originally approved for other purposes but are thought to also have an impact on cancer treatment. Many integrative oncologists and naturopathic physicians put great emphasis on supplements and OLDs. The range and variety of these recommendations are vast and bewildering.

Some recommendations make sense from the perspective of the TME and the hallmarks of cancer, and there is growing evidence that some cancer mechanisms can be affected. Natural products such as turmeric and green tea extracts seem to hit multiple hallmarks—they are pleiotropic. Combinations of herbs such as those used in traditional Chinese medicine would seem to be a good approach to influencing the TME and hallmarks of cancer if we only knew more about how to use them.

In 2019, Dr Keith Block, a prominent integrative oncologist in Chicago mentioned in Chapter 4, along with a large team of scientists from around the world, summarized what had been published by that point on natural product influences on the hallmarks of cancer. Those summaries were published in a special issue of the journal *Seminars in Cancer*.[31] The integrative oncologist Dr Dwight McKee published an updated review of over 40 natural products and their influence on the cancer hallmarks and the TME.[32] Several prominent oncologists have recently published summaries of the evidence for OLDs in cancer.[33] The Anticancer Fund, a European foundation, has been investing in research on OLDs for cancer management.[34] The process of moving old drugs into new uses is much faster and less expensive than developing an entirely new drug. The drugs still need to be studied for the new indication, but the many safety and toxicity studies have already been done. Profits from the use of OLDs, however, pale in comparison to new patent-protected drugs. We need more money directed to research on efficacy and use of OLDs.

Supplements and Natural Products

The challenge in using supplements and natural products is that the evidence usually comes from laboratory or animal models. Very few human clinical trials have been done to define their safety and efficacy, either alone or in combination. In the US, the regulation of dietary supplements is inadequate and lacks enforcement; the FDA investigates a product only if it gets a report of patient harm. Products often don't contain what they say they do; in some cases, they may contain toxic ingredients, adulterants, or contaminants. In addition to the complexities of getting quality products are issues of interaction and dosage.[35] Many herbal extracts are not well-absorbed and may not be getting into the TME even if they are ingested in large doses. For most supplements, we have insufficient research and remain uncertain on proper dosage or combinations. Finally, there are few studies looking at interactions of supplements with conventional treatments.

This is not to say that supplements should not be used. However, using supplements and natural products safely requires careful guidance and expertise—knowledge most oncologists don't have. Because of this many oncologists simply dismiss these products and tell patients not to use them. This unfortunately also dismisses what we do know about how they could positively affect the TME. Patients frequently use them anyway, often without telling their care team, creating a gap in communication and trust essential for good medical care. Patients who explore these areas on their own may end up getting poor-quality products, taking handfuls every day, and wasting money on dubious products. In the worst-case scenario, they may end up harming themselves through bad drug-supplement interactions.

As part of a whole person approach, oncology teams should guide patients on supplement use in a way that is nonjudgmental and evidence based. Fortunately, there are some guides to help oncology teams and people with cancer navigate this area. Memorial Sloan Kettering has put together an online supplement-drug interaction guide and evidence summaries that are a good place to start.[36] The NCI has an advisory panel (Dr Jonas is on this panel) that regularly reviews many of these supplements and provides summaries for both health professionals and patients of what is known about them.[37] Other reliable resources are the CAMCancer website, a European database;[38] and the Knowledge in Naturopathic Oncology Website (KNOW) database, a subscription-based searchable database on natural agents in cancer care. The KNOW database was created by OncANP, a professional organization for licensed Naturopathic Doctors (NDs) in North America.[39]

Off-Label Drugs

OLDs have a lot of potential for influencing 1 or more of the hallmarks of cancer. The production, dose (for the approved non-cancer indication), and safety profile of these drugs are usually well established, and the quality and absorption are defined. As mentioned earlier, little investment is going into exploring their role in cancer treatment, so optimal dosages and combinations aren't known. In addition, few OLDs actually kill cancer cells. Rather, they appear to influence 1 or more of the hallmarks and drivers of cancer. OLDs thus face the same challenge as supplements in knowing how much and in which combinations might be of benefit. Not surprisingly, the companies that supply combinations of OLDs recommend a wide variety of mixtures, even for the same cancer. Many patients are already taking 1 or more of these drugs for noncancer reasons, as prescribed by their primary care physicians and other specialists. Care teams need to be aware of the potential for interactions (both good and bad).

In complex situations, more information isn't always better. Determining the best approach even just for killing the cancer can often be confusing. Over the years, Jan got recommendations from various consultants for 7 different chemotherapy combinations and 4 types of surgery. She also had recommendations to use more than 15 OLDs and 30 natural product supplements. Each of these recommendations had some data (mostly laboratory, observational or pilot). She needed evidence-based guidance on which to use and when to not use them—a whole person approach to her care.

SUMMARY POINTS

- Cancer develops within a complex environment called the tumor microenvironment (TME).
- Detailed mechanisms of the TME have been described as the hallmarks of cancer biology.
- Immunity, metabolism and nutrition, and inflammation are major overarching mechanisms contributing to the hallmark processes.
- Macroenvironmental factors, including stress, nutrition, sleep, and other wellness factors influence these hallmarks.
- Off-label drugs (OLDs) and natural products may influence the hallmarks but are usually not sufficiently researched to know how to use them in cancer care.
- The biological science underlying cancer suggests practices that influence the tumor micro and macroenvironments optimize whole person care.

CHAPTER SIX

APPLYING SCIENCE IN WHOLE PERSON CARE

Knowledge about the biology of cancer means nothing unless oncology teams and people with cancer can access and use it alongside clinical data and evidence-based medicine. At the same time, we must remain cognizant about how little we know about any one person's cancer. Despite an explosion of cancer knowledge, as described in the previous chapter in this book, much of this knowledge is not used, paid for, or delivered to the patient. Our hope is that this book will help oncology teams change this situation.

Part of the delivery problem is operational and can be improved by redesigning how cancer care is managed and integrated. We discuss that in Chapter 15. However, oncology teams are often so overwhelmed with a focus on the immediate issues of the patient and the tumor staring them in the face that there is little time to address other factors or coordinate integration of care.[1] The evidence needed to address the tumor environment and the whole person doesn't get priority.

In addition, there is the ongoing challenge of taking aggregate data—as provided by evidence-based medicine—and applying it in predictive way to individuals, which is, of course, what patients and their care teams are looking to do. Known in statistics as the heterogeneous treatment effects (HTE) problem, new methods both as part of and beyond randomized studies are being explored.[2] Meanwhile, care teams must deal with this variability in response both when applying specific tumor treatments and whole person care approaches on a daily basis.

Finally, there is a lot we don't know about cancer and its healing. The body and person, including their disease and healing processes, are still largely a mystery. Scientists and clinicians are famous throughout the history of cancer for pushing the little they know to the limit (and beyond) without acknowledging that their knowledge sits in a sea of uncertainty. Because human beings generally don't like to admit we don't know, we apply the best evidence we have and often ignore the reality of our ignorance. This uncertainty may lead us to do more than what is required or beneficial. This is demonstrated in ASCO's Choosing Wisely campaign in oncology, a list of medical practices that are often used, even though the evidence shows they shouldn't be.[3]

In this chapter, we describe how to acknowledge and deal with both the scientific evidence and uncertainty. We believe it is important to employ not only critical thinking but also humility, listening, proper communication, expanded teams, and encouragement to patients to tap into their own intuition and decision-making.

EVIDENCE FOR WHAT AND FOR WHOM?

Dr Jonas has spent a good part of his career learning about, teaching, and applying research evidence in medicine. While Director of the Medical Research Fellowship at Walter Reed Army Institute of Research, he taught physicians how to think critically about research and scientific design, learn statistical methods, and understand the nuances of measurement. He oversaw and guided dozens of fellows in research and later led teams doing multiple types of research. While working for the Department of Defense, the NIH, and a WHO center, and advising the VA, he wrote, led, and taught research and the use of evidence in practice. He continues to teach about evidence-based medicine to residents and medical students at academic health centers around the world.

What he learned from decades of doing clinical and basic science is that the first factor to consider when defining what is "good" evidence is how that evidence will be used and by whom. Quality methods in doing the research are also important—but the research's intended use and application is just as important.

Truth and scientific validity are key to finding good evidence. False findings are especially damaging because, if believed, the information must be unlearned before valid information can be advanced. The rise of false information pushed by social media and magnified by AI has made establishment of quality science in the public sphere problematic. A 2023 Nobel Prize Summit called "Truth, Trust, and Hope," held in partnership with the National Academy of Sciences (NAS), discussed the growing challenges of using science to establish valid information.[4] In clinical medicine, having valid information is necessary but not sufficient to make it "good." Good evidence is only good when it is useful for those who need it. And the most important person who needs good evidence is the patient. Without knowing the patient, we can't find and apply good science properly. Jan's experience with her many cancers over the years illustrates this.

Scheduling, which was already a problem for Jan, became as onerous as the schedule of her oncologist. When pressed for time, she would sacrifice self-care to help with her grandchild or to go to medical appointments. However, when her mother needed her because her stepfather had died, Jan held off on getting treatment as her cancer recurred so she could help her mother. She created a self-styled version of whole person healing, but one that wasn't coordinated with her oncology team. In one situation, she sacrificed an important personal activity. In another, she sacrificed medical treatment.

How do we find research evidence to help guide us in the complex situations of whole person cancer care? First, let's review the basic types of evidence available. While many may know what types of research are available, we often don't clearly understand for what and whom they are most useful.

TYPES OF EVIDENCE

Whole person care calls on us to coordinate the use of evidence in an integrated way across the domains of patient and oncology teams. To do this, it is helpful to understand the types of evidence most often used in clinical decision-making. The figure below illustrates these types of evidence and which groups tend to need and prefer them. Dr Jonas calls this "The Evidence House." We will describe 4 of them.

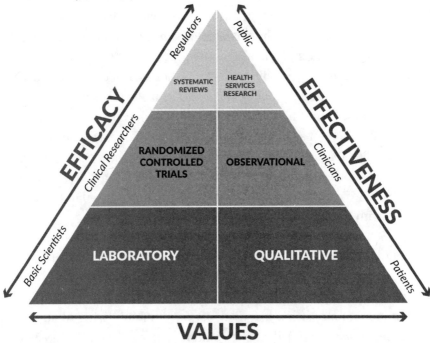

Figure 6.1 The Evidence House Model

This model shows a useful way to think about what types of evidence for clinical decision-making and for whom those types of evidence are most useful. Research types on the left side seek to explore cause and effect (attributional) evidence most valued by basic science, clinical researchers or regulators. Research types on the right side are looking for real-word effects most valued by patients, clinicians, and public health decisions.

Randomized Controlled Trials

Guidelines and FDA approvals are usually based on randomized control trials (RCTs), the optimal type of evidence for isolating cause and effect. RCTs are conducted by recruiting a carefully (and usually narrowly) selected group of patients and randomly assigning them to one treatment or another or to a control group, which is sometimes given a placebo (fake or mock) treatment. In RCTs of new cancer drugs, some patients are randomly assigned to get the usual treatment plus the new drug; the others get usual treatment and a placebo. If the study is double-blinded, the patients and clinician/researchers don't know who is getting what treatment until the study is completed. Whether blinded or not, randomization evens out the starting point for all patients and increases the ability to detect whether a new treatment is beneficial or not. Properly conducted RCTs have a type of rigor called internal validity. As important as RCTs are, they also have limitations, usually around external validity, or generalizability.

Only a small minority (about 5%) of patients ever enter randomized controlled trials. The reasons are complex but a major one is that to control and isolate the specific effects being tested, a narrow group of similar patients must be recruited. In addition, many patients don't want to be part of an "experiment" even if it is their best chance of getting something that may work better than the standard. Patients that participate in RCTs represent a subgroup of all people with that particular cancer, but study results are later applied in the complex and changing real world, where the target population is broader and more diverse. In practice, generalizing the results to individual patients is often a challenge and limitation of RCTs.

RCTs are designed mainly for use in population-based guidelines and for regulatory approval by the FDA to determine if a specific treatment or drug causes a specific outcome. This is called attribution. Thus, data from RCTs are most useful for those decision-makers.

Observational Studies

Large observational studies, or epidemiological studies, don't randomize people into separate arms that receive different treatments. Instead, they try to mathematically sort out what might be producing the effects by looking at large groups of people already receiving different treatments. Observational studies are more generalizable because they include a broad variety of patients. The disadvantage is that we can't know for sure whether the treatment analyzed is the one producing the effect. Many factors that influence cancer coexist, and this can confound the analysis of any one variable and confuse us on whether to believe in the findings. These studies are used when randomization isn't possible, such as studies on the impact of smoking, alcohol, diet, and behavior on cancer risk and treatment. They give us probabilities in a messy world. If the intervention is safe and low cost, observational studies may be sufficient to recommend and use an approach. This is often the type of information needed for cancer teams and patients in usual practice looking to attain whole person care. Many of the wellness approaches described in Chapters 4 and 12 fall into this category because they are low risk. Patients and clinicians need this type of research to get an idea of the likelihood that benefit, more than harm, will occur in noncontrolled conditions, such as in regular practice.

Basic Science

Basic science research usually involves studying cells and animal models. It's the source for much of our detailed understanding of the tumor microenvironment and the hallmarks of cancer discussed in the previous chapter. This type of research helps us understand mechanisms at the cellular or molecular level, but the information often falls apart when tested in the real world of complex human beings. As one of Dr Jonas's research mentors pointed out, "Any cancer can be cured in mice." Many a company (and patient) has discovered that cures in test tubes and lab mice don't often translate into cures for human beings. Still, we draw on this information when trying to make decisions amid uncertainty or when the guideline-approved approaches stop working.

The vast complexity of the cancer process now shows that even in the same patient and the same tumor, the biology may have tremendous variation. Jan's tumor may have started with a specific genetic inheritance, mutation, or injury; but its growth and progression were a dance of cat and mouse between the cancer cells, the microenvironment and macroenvironment around the cells, her behavior, and her engagement with the oncology team. Personalized care requires us to engage the art of medicine while playing our best cards with cutting-edge science. This dynamic dance can't be easily captured in guidelines or one type of evidence. It requires the integration of data, time, and intuition.

Qualitative Research

Qualitative research is the systematic documentation of subjective aspects of a topic under study. This is the most overlooked type of evidence because it involves intuition. Patients need to feel intuitively that the approaches they are using have been successful in people that look, feel and think like them. This need should not be taken lightly by the oncology team. People with cancer need to hear from others who they can identify with and learn their stories. Drug companies and others frequently use patient anecdotes for marketing purposes, but these stories leave out crucial information. The data from the stories can turn into good qualitative information if collected properly and analyzed rigorously. Qualitative research provides evidence for better understanding of what matters to patients, an important component of whole person care. It can help us see what we're missing in our knowledge and where we can fill in those gaps with other types of research.

USING THE EVIDENCE: THE FOUR Ps

How do we use these different types of research evidence in practice? Each has different uses for decision-making. Regulators look for proof of cause and effect in controlled settings from RCTs. Practitioners often use observational research to look for the probability of benefit or harm. Patients may be looking for stories of patients like themselves in qualitative terms, and people who want to "do everything" may dive into basic research when trying to understand cancer mechanisms and care.

No one type of research is inherently better than another when done well and used correctly. Determining what's good for a patient may draw on some or all of them. Good evidence isn't a hierarchy. As the philosopher of science Henri Poincaré said, "Science is built of facts the way a house is built of bricks: but an accumulation of facts is no more science than a pile of bricks is a house."[5]

Dealing with all the evidence and information needed for whole person care is always a challenge. How do we think about the different types of evidence? How can we better use them in day-to-day practice? Evidence comes basically in 3 buckets: the clearly known, the partially known, and the unknown. Unfortunately, at any given time the biggest of these buckets is usually the last bucket, the unknown.

A useful framework for thinking about how to use evidence is called the Four Ps.

Protect

The first P is to protect. The Hippocratic Oath tells us "First, do no harm." But harm sometimes must be inflicted to heal; in the treatment of cancer, the harm can sometimes be quite extensive. However, harm can come in many forms: direct harm delivered through the treatments; harm that occurs from not treating the disease; harm from interactions of things that when given alone are benign; harm from nocebo effects due to incorrect beliefs and bad communication, and harm from financial toxicity. We first need to make sure we are protecting patients as much as possible from all these types of harm.

Permit

The second P is to permit. Patients often want to engage in their own treatment, go outside standard recommendations, and "do everything" they can to treat the cancer and prevent recurrence—even if those approaches don't have full evidence for safety and efficacy.

They may or may not seek permission from oncologists to use these treatments. In discussing treatment options with patients, explore the risk, benefit, and evidence underlying various approaches. We know that empowerment and the placebo effect are powerful tools for helping patients engage in treatment and stimulate their own healing. If an approach isn't harmful but empowers the patient in their own healing journey, that practice may be a reasonable one to consider from the patient point of view. Patients may not expect you to provide an unorthodox treatment, but they're often looking for the team's openness to pursue it. Not everything can be proven through an RCT efficacy study. But if an approach isn't harmful, then room for its use should be explored.

Promote

The third P is promote. If a practice has been proven and is now recommended in guidelines, we should consider promoting it and make an effort to provide that service. Conversely, when the evidence demonstrates that a practice isn't beneficial, then we should consider not recommending or doing it. The latter is the principle behind ASCO's Choosing Wisely and doing less.

Partner

The fourth P is to partner with the patient and their extended care team. A whole person case conference is an example of how to do that formally (more on this later). Partnering can also be done informally and continuously if a foundation of access and trust is built between the patient, the oncologist, and the larger team. That trust rests on the shared intention for optimal health and life, and it is delivered through respect, listening, and compassion.

THE COMPLEXITY OF USING SCIENCE

Applying all the evidence that has accumulated in guidelines, ongoing science, and other research on cancer care is a challenging task. In primary medical care, there aren't nearly enough hours in the day to do everything that's recommended. The same is true in cancer care. Unless we come up with more efficient delivery systems, a lot of good science goes by the wayside. Add to that the needs of whole person care, and many oncologists and their teams focus on satisfying the metrics being tracked, stick to primarily killing the cancer, and try to stay up to date with what science they can.

For Jan, the desired outcomes from her 2 worlds—what matters and what's the matter—were rarely discussed. The oncology teams wanted to implement a rigorous series of combination chemotherapies for her breast cancer that would increase her chances of 5-year disease free survival by 7%. Jan wanted to improve her chances, but she also wanted the time and energy to help take care of her newborn grandson. She wanted to reduce both the time involved in treatments and her fatigue. Activities such as acupuncture (which helped Jan's energy) were often put aside for other goals. No one asked Jan if a 7% gain was worth the sacrifice of her own goals, her self-care, and the side effects. No one asked if there were logistical and navigational approaches that could help her accomplish them all. She had to bring in her own advocate and advocate for herself for that to happen.

In whole person care, these types of discussions are recommended as a standard part of shared decision-making (SDM). This approach of SDM and the topic of advocacy were both discussed in Chapter 2. Now we discuss ways to apply the science of whole person care in practice, ways that involve SDM and patient advocates.

The Person-Centered Case Conference

Teams are used to having huddles, tumor boards, and other forms of case-based conferences. We recommend reorganizing and renaming tumor boards into "person-centered care meetings" or, shorter, "care planning meetings" that get input about and make time to focus on what matters to the person ahead of the meeting, so that it can be shared with the larger team making medical recommendations. This allows what matters, and any lifestyle factors that are already an issue, to be identified as care planning proceeds. Many times, multidisciplinary tumor boards include people who can help but who have not yet met the patient to do so.

Sharing information directly from a patient in such a meeting can expedite care. A well-written editorial in *JCO Oncology Practice* provides further support in renaming tumor boards, should you be interested to see how it may assist a move to whole person care planning at your institution.[6] If we keep talking the way we always have, about patients (rather than people), about noncompliance (rather than choice), and about tumors (rather than people) things will not change as rapidly as we might hope.

As an example, IOLC members from northern Virginia's Inova Schar Cancer Institute, did this by inviting newly diagnosed patients with gastrointestinal (GI) malignancies to answer a few HOPE questions before the conference via EPIC's MyChart. In a newly termed "GI care planning meeting," patient answers to HOPE questions were shown on an intro slide (made by the team social worker) before the usual multidisciplinary slides shared from radiology, pathology, and the like. Inova's physician-social worker team co-led by Jennifer Bires, LCSW, Executive Director of Life with Cancer (LWC) and Patient Experience for the Inova Schar Cancer Institute, ensures patients have access to a LWC therapist, detailed as part of the multidisciplinary care planning process, to provide up front and specific focus on crisis intervention, adjustment to illness and evidence-based support for nonpharmacological management of symptoms. Below are examples of patients' sharing within the GI care planning meeting.

From a 46-year-old married mother of two (colon cancer): Lifestyle: walks, yardwork; What You Should Know About the Patient: "I am very proactive and plan to work as hard as possible to beat this cancer. If you could help me get appointments and procedures set up as speedily as possible, that would make me the most happy. I think time is of the essence."

From a 71-year-old man with liver cancer: Lifestyle: hiking/ spending time with grandkids, currently experiencing lack of energy, anticipatory worry about medical condition and poor sleep hygiene; What You Should Know About the Patient: "I feel fortunate to have lived a healthy life. I am a person of faith and I do not have an urge to extend life simply to avoid death."

These patients are depicted in more than 1 dimension, and as more than the abnormal scans and cells otherwise depicted to teams as "the case." Recommendations for care become more useful if a person's needs are met early on; this tweak to a usual tumor board format allowed whole person care to begin right away at Inova.

Although similar in structure, a whole person case conference isn't the same as the care planning meeting discussed previously. Here is an example of one arranged to be held virtually to include a person with complex medical needs, Sarah. Sarah had complex regional pain syndrome (CRPS), a chronic condition often initiated by surgery or other injuries. When she was diagnosed with node-positive triple negative breast cancer, surgery was recommended. Sarah was deeply concerned about the pain consequences surgery might induce. She had had prolonged CRPS flares from surgery before. She and her patient advocate gathered a team of advisers, including her primary oncologist at a major academic center and outside consultants.

They all met (virtually), Sarah included, for a person-centered case conference and devised a plan for a combination of chemotherapy and immunotherapy to shrink her tumor. This would be followed by cryotherapy under hypnosis. As part of the treatment plan, Sarah engaged in lifestyle and behavioral factors to reduce chronic inflammation. Low-dose steroids were added when the immunotherapy made autoimmune processes flare up. The pain from this was successfully treated with Reiki. She also engaged in meditation, swimming, and acupuncture and took selected supplements during treatment. The plan worked remarkably to improve her wellbeing and reduce both the tumor and her pain. Thankfully, the cryotherapy didn't aggravate her CRPS. Such is the power of a person-centered case conference with an appropriately trained and empowered patient advocate, and with an engaged patient.

Oncologists do not have to be the formal care advocate or run the whole person aspect of such case conferences. Yet oncologists do have an important leadership role in whole person care. By encouraging patients to get involved in their own care, and providing shared space and authority for patient advocates, and others on the care team, they can fully participate in developing a whole person care plan.[7] A recent survey by IQVIA[8] showed that the most important motivator for patients to become engaged in whole person care is the support and recommendation of their oncologist.[9]

DOING LESS

By the time Jan had a recurrence of ovarian cancer, she felt she was doing too many things, both mainstream and integrative, to treat it. This was impinging on one of her main goals—spending time with her grandchildren and friends and traveling with and caring for her family. She decided to take stock and stop some parts of her treatment.

In practice, oncology teams get into information overload because we keep adding on things to do, but rarely take things away. However, the application of good evidence goes both ways. Often, research points to things that have long been part of practice but should no longer be done. Periodically reviewing what you and your team are doing, with the specific intent of applying a Choosing Wisely-type view to processes and then stopping some that don't bring value, is a good practice.

On the complementary medicine side, many come in taking handfuls of supplements several times a day, sometimes at substantial cost as noted in Chapter 5. Helping patients sort through those substances with the goal of removing or adjusting them can be helpful. Less can be more. In Jan's case, integrative oncology practitioners recommended quercetin, high-dose vitamin C, alpha-lipoic acid, curcumin, resveratrol, and mushroom extracts. The recommendations were often based on genetic markers found in her tumor. When her cancers recurred or progressed, however, it was time to stop some of those treatments.

Patients may want to try multiple things at once, whereas most oncologists prefer to provide a single treatment and use it until it fails. The simultaneous approach may bring comfort to the patient that they are being proactive, but it quickly becomes confusing when a supplement or complementary treatment seems to work—or when it doesn't or creates interactions and side effects. The sequential approach has the benefit of determining whether a treatment is working or not. When treatments are toxic, however, they may exhaust the person with cancer, sometimes to the point of abandoning conventional therapy or giving up prematurely.

Other approaches to doing less require more research but are promising for greater patient comfort. These include low-dose combination chemotherapies, chemotherapy delivered in a cyclical or continuously infused manner, and timing with biological cycles (chronotropic chemotherapy). Fewer lifestyle interventions, or more carefully timed ones, might also be beneficial. There is early evidence for the possible benefit of fasting before chemo.[10] Such approaches need more research before they're ready for routine use, but patients will ask about them or try them, sometimes without informing the care team. Care teams can prepare to address them with patients by using the 4P principles.

AVOIDING THE NOCEBO EFFECT

Then there is the need to avoid harm from even harmless interventions or what is sometimes called the nocebo effect. Recommending treatments without evidence is the first harm, as patients then may go off on a wild goose chase with the "toxicities" of time, finances, and false hope. Then there is the concern of causing harm through the way we communicate the evidence. Saying to a patient that "you" as an individual person will fall into 1 of 2 groups—those that will live on or those to die of the disease—is not a prediction with less than 100% accuracy. Applying probability data to an individual is not only an improper use of science and statistics, but it also risks harming them or giving them false hope.[11] No one can make infallible predictions about how an individual patient will do. When prognostic proclamations come from an authority, they can become especially harmful, producing a nocebo effect. This is like what shamans call a "curse,"—an expectation of harm. Extensive research (mostly outside of oncology) on the placebo and nocebo effect shows that expectation and ritual in a medical setting can produce either negative or positive effects—both psychological and physiological.[12]

Even informed consent, a requirement before procedures and chemotherapy or when participating in a clinical trial, has been shown to increase the rate of symptoms experienced by patients, both objective and subjective. In one study, for example, patients' negative expectations of side effects from endocrine therapy for breast cancer over a 2-year period increased those side effects (and others).[13] The authority of the oncologist and the vulnerability of the cancer patient enhance these effects almost as if they were under hypnosis.[14] Oncology teams can train team members in proper language and how to communicate about the science of cancer, the nature of research, and their implications for prognosis and the effects of treatments, both adverse and beneficial.

THE SEA OF UNCERTAINTY

Based on what we see historically, we can surmise that the traditional view in oncology was most often a simple, direct, and linear one, which may look, for example, like the shortest path between 2 points. If we suggest that point A is diagnosis and point B is treatment, the shortest path from one to the other is a straight line. If we suggest point A and point B are instances in time, the faster we move on the path between, the faster we arrive. If point A is cancer and point B is no cancer, you end up with treatments such as the Halstead surgery that do not take into account the whole. But we know now that cancer does not work that way. Rapid regression of cancer does not always translate into longer survival, yet we still want to see the cancer gone as quickly as possible.

Oncology sits in a sea of uncertainties, within the larger uncertain field of medicine. A place to see this uncertainty is in the typical Kaplan-Meier (KM) survival curves so often used to show that one cancer treatment modality is definitively better than another.

— **New Treatment** — **Standard Care**

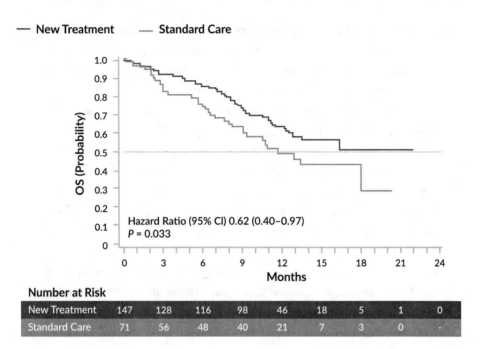

Figure 6.2 Kaplan-Meier Curve for Overall Survival

This is an example of how new cancer treatment data are presented. Two treatments being compared are a new treatment and placebo or standard care. The separation between the curves illustrates the better treatment (higher curve). The rapid drop off in survival illustrates the ocean of ignorance we all swim in, still.

The figure shows a typical KM graph for a new "breakthrough" treatment for advanced cancer. In this graph 100% of patients start out alive. Then there is a rapid drop off in survival over a period (here it is 24 months). The new treatment works better than standard of care if the curves begin to separate, with the top curve being the better one depicting the group with better survival, and this becomes the preferred treatment. But the uncertainty is staring us in the face as both curves drop off rapidly with few survivors (less than 20%) in the end. The benefit (calculated as a "hazard ratio") can look large if relative differences are calculated between treatments while the few survivors in the end show that uncertainty dominates the entire process. Even using the "break-through" treatment represented by the top curve only 5 of 147 patients are alive at 18 months—but this is 2 more than usual care. Communicating this information to a patient is complicated. We try to use words like "curable" and "treatable" carefully, although people may not understand what we mean by them.

Asking a patient to repeat their understanding of what the treatment is supposed to do, for example, before they sign the informed consent for a treatment, can go a long way to making sure the person received the message we were trying to send and has fully consented to it. Even when the person with cancer understands what we mean, uncertainty remains. Will the patient in front of you be in that percent still alive "on the curve" at end of the study? Of course, if they are, their individual survival is 100%. Moreover, the result represents only one outcome and, depending on the patient, may not be the most important one.

HUMILITY: THE RESPONSE TO UNCERTAINTY

While his most famous book is the previously mentioned *Emperor of All Maladies*, Dr Siddhartha Mukherjee is also the author of a lesser-known book, *The Laws of Medicine: Field Notes from an Uncertain Science*.[15] It discusses the uncertainty of science in medical decision-making, especially cancer treatment. We can understand why that book remains less widely read. Facing uncertainty is uncomfortable. The discomfort that arises when we're faced with uncertainty despite all our science introduces the topic of mystery. In medicine and nursing, we have little room for consideration of this space we all wander through, whether as patients ourselves or in caring for people with cancer. Consider how you may "know" what led to a certain outcome when you or a loved one weren't well, or how you ascribe meaning to your own experiences of healing. In both scenarios, you may find yourself in a place of mystery and awe. We have all heard stories from patients who "knew" something was not right in their body. This led them to push for more care and diagnostics, and eventually brought them to our doors in cancer care. Jan asked for her ovaries to be removed even while there were no guidelines to do so. That is how her ovarian cancer was caught early.

AI will not solve the uncertainty dilemma. The greatest AI engine is the patient's own intuition—if it can be properly nurtured and guided with evidence. Patients frequently know more about what's going on with their bodies than they can articulate, or that care teams have time to hear. Consciously or not, people with cancer integrate their own intuition into their decision-making. They may get some of their clearest insights while meditating or engaging in a spiritual practice. Or in a dream. It may also happen while doing something that frees the mind for a few moments— gardening or even washing the dishes. When people relax and release their fears, clarity often emerges.

Science and good evidence are crucial for good care. But for whole person care to occur, many other factors about what matters in life must come into play. The oncology team can strive to culti-vate intuition and patient preference and weave this with science. This doesn't mean the team does everything the patient wants. It means that humility, time, and trust in the process are the only ways to honestly face the vast unknown in which we all swim.

SUMMARY POINTS

- Good evidence using quality science is one of the great advances in modern medicine.

- What makes evidence "good" in patient care is that it is patient-relevant, rigorously done and ready for real-time, real-world use.

- Different types of evidence are provided by different types of research and for different purposes. One type of research design is not inherently more important than all others for all purposes.

- Even with good science, there is always a large amount of uncertainty in a particular situation.

- Having a patient champion or advocate and using case conferences designed to include the patient voice are useful steps in the implementation of whole person care.

- Learning how to communicate about evidence in a way that avoids the nocebo effect can prevent harm.

- The rational (science) and the nonrational (intuition) both have a place in decision-making.

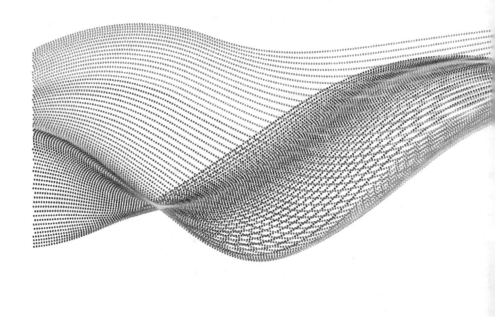

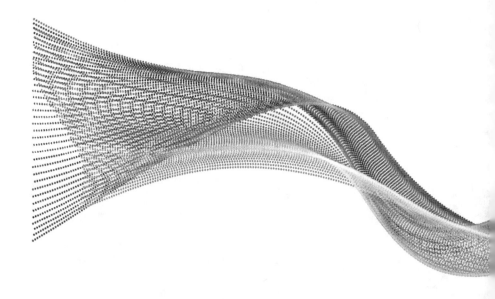

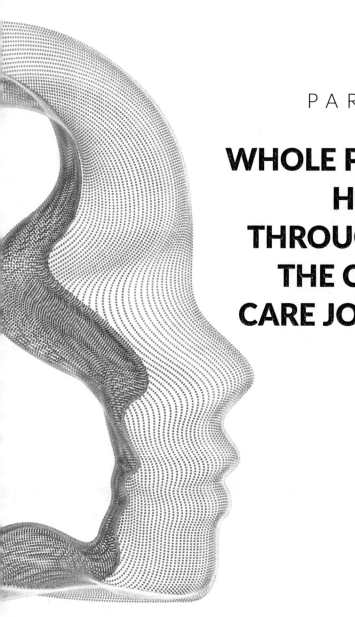

PART TWO

WHOLE PERSON HEALING THROUGHOUT THE CANCER CARE JOURNEY

CHAPTER SEVEN

DIAGNOSIS

When we meet someone for the first time following diagnosis, cancer is a living entity in the room, an invader in the person's body. Some may later find it possible to befriend the invader, transmuting it into a visiting professor in the school of life, but not most. And not now. At diagnosis, first there is fear, or denial, or anger, or any other "unexpected visitor" as found in Rumi's famous poem, "The Guest House." It is here, in this place of many visitors, where we do our work.

At diagnosis, whether we acknowledge it or not, a lot is going on for both team and patient. All of us face some degree of anxiety over death, uncertainty, and loss. When Dr Jonas's wife was diagnosed with breast cancer, they met in a parking lot, held each other and cried. "How will we tell the kids?" was her first question. In fact, she went more than 25 years after treatment without cancer, but there was no way to know that at the time. Even after 25 years, the fear and grief remain and must be faced, albeit altered by time. Each patient is unique. Getting to know them, their circumstances, and what matters most to them early on pays off later in trust, relationships, shared decision-making and better overall care.

Working in oncology gives us familiarity with this variable terrain. We come to know some diagnoses or circumstances as somehow better and easier to befriend than others, because they're largely survivable or, as in the case of ductal carcinoma *in situ* (DCIS), sometimes described as "not even cancer." (Best not to say that to someone in the middle of treatment, or maybe ever.) Our teams' knowledge of cancer as either a nuisance or a formidable foe comes at a price. As much as our learning can guide a person with cancer through the first steps following diagnosis, we can lose sight of what it may look like from their perspective. When we become desensitized, we forget that we also face pain, suffering, and eventual mortality. We may fail to see that the person in front of us is untethered and drifting upon mortal fear, or clear eyed and sanguine, even in the face of their mortality.[1] If we can start without assumptions, we more easily remember that we do not know, but need to find out, what any one person wants or is experiencing at the time of diagnosis (or after). Considering this, in this chapter we look at how whole person care concepts can inform care starting from diagnosis.

TISSUE IS THE ISSUE (AND WAITING IS THE WORST)

Biopsy, or having needles stuck into body parts, is noxious at best and dehumanizing at worst. Our colleagues in surgery and radiology do amazing things to get the tissue that allows for diagnosis and staging to occur and a treatment plan to develop. Sometimes, no further treatment is indicated.

For the person with suspected cancer, the diagnostic process is usually rife with anxiety. It's tied to anticipation of pain and potential confirmation of the diagnosis—or the anticipation of more procedures and even more uncertainty if diagnosis remains elusive. The required signing of consent documents, with their frightening lists of possible complications—including death—can create anxiety even before the actual procedure. When the documents are presented without sensitivity, this can trigger the nocebo effect as discussed in other chapters.

And then, the waiting for test results begins. Pathology reports and the increasingly complex testing required to deliver person-alized cancer therapy don't materialize immediately. The void of the waiting period fills most easily with anxiety. While the initial diagnosis is perhaps not the time to introduce mindfulness as a coping skill, it can buffer the impact of anxiety later on.[2]

As Tom Petty wrote, "The waiting is the hardest part." During this high-anxiety period for patients and their loved ones, care teams can offer whatever help and resources they can, including support resources found in their hospital system or cancer center.[3] In lessening the waiting for results of staging scans and biopsies, electronic patient portals are a double-edged sword; teams with built-in processes to convey results within context as soon as humanly possible in fact lessen, but do not resolve, people's anxi-ety at diagnosis.

Modalities such as mindfulness, music therapy, guided imag-ery, virtual reality, or other forms of relaxation techniques, could be offered earlier, sooner, and in your waiting room—or taught to patients online or through free or low-cost apps. A plethora of studies suggests safe and effective interventions to quell anxiety in people with cancer. Why wait to introduce nonpharmacologic modalities that address quality of life and reduce anxiety? Your teams are experts in the resources offered by your institution and community. A group brainstorm on what best fits your practice's and your population's needs can help everyone become more aware of available and appropriate resources. See Chapter 12 for more on effective interventions.

Consider community-based ties that can make your waiting room a healing space. Perhaps a local musician or artist, possibly also a past patient, is looking to give back in some way. Volunteers can fill gaps where anxiety lingers, like in waiting rooms stifled as much by dread-filled quiet as by TV news (which usually adds to anxiety these days). It doesn't take a well-designed clinical trial to tell us that people diagnosed with cancer come to us already suffering. But it does take empathy and awareness of these feel-ings, allowing us to imagine what it is like to be on the other side of diagnosis, to provide the kind of care we know can make a difference.

LIVING THINGS AFFIRM LIFE

If you don't have access yet to a very different type of AI in your workplace, AAI (animal assisted intervention), see if it would be a fit. We're not suggesting a bone marrow transplant unit should be on the list for pet therapy, but as we look for ways to decrease distress at a person's intake (or any) appointment following diagnosis, AAI could help. For people who gravitate to animals, the presence of another living, loving thing can counter fear, if only for a moment. That moment, acknowledging the sweetness of a canine or touching the softness of a furry coat, becomes a thread in the memory of the medical encounter. If you need more than your own lived experience to consider the benefit of AAI in oncology, a systematic review of the literature covering 32 studies showed, "AAIs generally have a neutral, sometimes positive, association with the physiological and psychological endpoints of interest. Specifically, oxygen saturation increased, quality of life improved, perceived satisfaction with AAI was high, and depression and other negative mood states decreased among research participants. Most, if not all, other variables—both physiological (for example, heart rate, blood pressure, respiration rate, and cortisol) and psychological (for example, anxiety, distress, hostility, self-perceived health, and quality of life)—investigated across studies showed no significant changes with AAI."[4]

AAIs may or may not be right for your clinic. But if you consider what it means to be a living thing among other living things, you may find there is a real benefit. And a benefit for your patients translates to a benefit for their caregivers and the larger team. If AAI is of interest, allowing someone on your team to take this on as a "pet project" may be just the thing to improve morale during this time of unprecedented burnout. For those coming in for care and at the time of diagnosis, unscripted AAI could be a positive experience. If this is a bridge too far, there is always the possibility of a living plant (or deepfake) strategically placed in our otherwise sterile environment to allow a glimpse of life to take up some space, and to counter the death thoughts running underground. Just be sure to have someone dust off the foliage once in a while!

FEAR: SAY MY NAME

Getting to a diagnosis names the invader in very specific terms. There's also a benefit to naming the related fear. This is where team social workers and behavioral health specialists, therapists and counselors make impact. Kind words shared at the front desk check in can also ameliorate fear.[5] Selecting and training front office workers in remembering names, and responding with patience, kindness, and listening goes a long way in helping many patients feel comfortable. Jan switched practices on at least one occasion because of the front office staff's low social and emotional capacity; she was sure it reflected on the leadership in the clinic. Many team members in cancer care provide empathetic support, yet time for dedicated psychosocial support is not always available to the person at diagnosis intake.

Oncologist as Gatekeeper

When it comes to ameliorating fear, the oncologist has a gatekeeping function that places a burden squarely in their lap. At the first visit, they strive to provide information, answering questions to keep uncertainty at bay. At this meeting there is data to share, evidence to reassure, truth to tell when it comes to prognosis and to treatment—if the person wants it. Teams spend a lot of mental energy assessing what people may want, most often tacitly and only sometimes by asking directly, which takes time.

The first visit following diagnosis is intense for both doctor and patient. The person with cancer or their loved ones may have looked up general statistics online. Most don't know how to interpret group probability data and think the 5-year survival numbers seal their personal fate. This error should be corrected at the first meeting with education and illustration of what population data really mean. It takes time and practice to deliver this information in an understandable and reassuring way. If the prognosis is particularly dire, the visit can provoke anxiety—sharing and receiving such information is very difficult. White-knuckling through this internal discomfort can become a routine, for team members, patients, and caregivers alike.

Among the team members, anxieties may sublimate. Sublimation is very useful to the organizations that house our care teams, as immersion in work, a seemingly healthy outlet, can become a tendency toward overwork. Over time, teams may do more with less, even without being asked! Sound familiar? If we address and acknowledge burnout and moral injury, both personal and systemic, we can reduce their impact.

A WORD ON BURNOUT

More than 2 decades' worth of publications describe the scope of burnout in cancer care. Incidence is estimated as being in the 30 to 50% range.[6,7,8] There is a high likelihood you or someone on your team has experienced burnout directly. If not to the point of burnout, the stress of cancer care will often reduce teams' wellbeing if not acknowledged, addressed, and managed directly.

Dr McManamon recounts her own experience of burnout from overwork during a time as solo oncologist in community-based practice. She recalls:

> I know the phenomenon as a lived experience with clear consequences for care, but knowing isn't always doing. In my experience of burnout, people become work. There is no access to joy. Perfectionistic tendencies lead to negative bias and short-fused response to the inevitable frustrations inherent in clinical care. In the end, I learned there is no way to provide whole person care without honoring the wholeness of the people doing the caring, whatever role they play on the team—including my own wholeness. I think it's important to share that

this period of burnout occurred for me years after I knew (and had been teaching) Dr Rachel Remen's work as known from courses such as The Healer's Art™. This program is offered in more than half of all US medical schools and internationally as an inoculation of sorts against burnout. Well before this, I had been co-director of the course at my alma mater, the Uniformed Services University of the Health Sciences, for 7 years! It doesn't matter if you know about burnout. If circumstances are right (read: wrong), you can still know burnout very up-close and personal. Educational programming from the Remen Institute for the Study of Health and Illness[9] strengthens individuals' skills in finding meaning in our work. It helps us realize that we, in our wholeness, are what patients and their caregivers need, just as much as they need our expertise. Curing is one thing and not always possible, but healing is always available, as becomes apparent to those who participate in the Healer's Art. Coming out of burnout (in this case only because I got a vacation and a work partner), I increasingly embraced my wholeness in providing care. But I also know I am just as vulnerable as I ever was when expectations are impossible to satisfy, whether external/institutional or my own unrealistic fantasy of how my cancer care should look. I now know better how to ask for help, and how to accept it, even if this is still hard for me (as I suspect it may be for you). In real-time, I again experience joy in practice and see, as you likely do, the privilege we have in taking care of people facing cancer. But I also know that I must push back when things don't make sense. I am more activated to support my teammates and do so more actively. I think often of what my mom used to say, ironically,

when I would complain to her (as a younger physician, at that time in the military and under a
service obligation), "What are they going to do, fire
you?" It helps to realize what (and who) actually
leads to the provision of the safest and best care
for our patients. In oncology, unless you are doing
something unquestionably wrong, you are probably about to do something right when it comes to
self-care and inroads to whole person care.

THE BEST CARE IS THE SAFEST CARE

And what about the best care for our patients? We all want them to
feel safe enough to ask the necessary questions at the first meeting
and beyond. But as they may have waited some time for their intake
appointment, they are aware of the time crunch and workforce
shortage issues. People sometimes hold back on asking questions,
not just out of an initial overwhelm but also out of respect for our
time (or lack thereof).

We need to give signals from the start that the oncology office
is a safe place to ask questions; acknowledging fear helps create the
safe space. Pausing, listening, sitting down, facing the patient and
not the computer screen, asking if they have questions about issues
one at a time instead of in a blanket statement-question (actually
made of many rapid-fire questions in a row), and clear direction
on how to contact the team after they leave the visit are all signs
that you're ready to hear anything from them. Adding something
as open-ended as, "What else?" when looking to conclude an initial
visit can help. At an initial meeting, use all your skills—and maybe
try out some new approaches—to let your patient know you are
there for them in a space of learning and moving forward together.
Listening brings a great gift of healing.

Nobody likes to be the bearer of bad news, but in oncology it's
part of the job. Just as it can be powerful to name an emotion in
our personal lives and diffuse its hold on us, the same applies in
our work lives. When someone at work seems upset, we're taught

it's OK to say, "You seem really upset." The person will typically and emphatically agree, "Yes, I'm upset!" and they may go into all the reasons why. Or they may state what they're really feeling, "No, I'm not upset. I'm furious!" Lines of communication open when an emotion is named. It draws the sentiment out into a place where we can objectively examine it together. Could it be that just by calling out the fear at diagnosis and stating its presence, whether a patient's or your own, we are better able to help the patient? Acknowledging our own anxiety in some useful way before giving bad news could be as simple as writing down any concerns to get them out (even if no one else will ever see them). Even simpler, allow yourself a moment to feel whatever is present, with hand on door handle or during hand hygiene (both good prompts), then taking a deep breath before entering into the encounter. Your breath is always with you and hand hygiene is always required. Simple acknowledgments such as these allow cultivation of self-awareness within the natural workflow, and the benefit-to-risk ratio is high. Acknowledging that we all may find freedom in living through, rather than sublimating, feelings is a move forward in whole person care—yours and theirs.

To name fear as common in the experience of those newly diagnosed with cancer, someone from the team might communicate to the person preintake, "We're here to support you as you face this new diagnosis. This can be a scary time, and we understand you may be feeling anxiety or fear right now. We want you to know we'll be inviting you to discuss this up front, to help answer the questions we can about the unknown future. We are here to walk through this journey with you. We need your full participation and if, at any time, you feel we have gotten off track from what you need, we invite you to let us know so we can do the best to care for you."

Or, more simply, an oncologist can reassure at intake, "Fear is a normal part of the experience at the time of a cancer diagnosis. If you're feeling fear, it's normal. We welcome you to talk about how you are feeling." Then be quiet, allow silence, and see how it goes. You may learn the person accepts their fear and is capable of moving forward with it. You may learn the person is paralyzed by it, not sleeping, or isolating to cope. Or you may learn they fall somewhere in between. No matter what the fear response is, you'll be learning about the person in front of you. That knowledge will inform the care you and your team provide.

Creating a safe psychological space for your patient at that first visit is priceless. It sets you both on the path of mutual trust from the start. And it occurs in small ways, such as allowing silence (to give the person time to absorb and/or respond to what you have said), being present with emotion (possibly gently inquiring what they're thinking or feeling), and taking cues from patients and caregivers as to what they need in the moment.

PRACTICE

Training is helpful. Practice is essential. For many of us, communication skills are not automatic. Health care education rarely teaches us how to do this. You may need to try new ways of being and new lines of questioning. You may have to keep doing this until you feel comfortable, sense more comfort in your patients, or both. Progress allows us to learn from the inevitable mistakes we are certain to make in practice. As mentioned earlier, when Dr Jonas's wife was first diagnosed with breast cancer, her doctor wanted to rush her to surgery. Dr Jonas shares further:

> The first cancer surgeon rushed the conversation, and his fear spilled over and fed our fear. We consulted a second surgeon who exuded warmth, patience, and kindness. He named our fear right up front, and we both felt much of our anxiety melt away. I doubt the amount of time spent in these 2 visits were much different, but the impact and aftermath were huge. You could hear the breathing relax and deepen in the room. Afterward, we enjoyed a dinner out for the first time in weeks. We then more clearly thought through our needs and the plan.

Naming emotions deepens relationships in a way that allows for better care throughout the journey. For oncology care providers—who are people too—naming emotions humanizes us to ourselves in a vast field of potential suffering. Cultivating an ability to create a safe space, you wordlessly say to your patients, "I see you. I am here for you."

We can also not do that. We can distance ourselves and provide just the facts. We can answer questions to the best of our ability, as we strive to do already. But we may miss something in the sterility of numbers lined up defensively in the evolving diagnostic landscape—being a living person in the presence of another living person, together.

If naming emotions and being a human being at work sounds scary (it can be), don't go it alone. Make sure to find at least one teammate to debrief with when you try something new. At work these days, with all the literal masking we've endured, no one knows how you really feel unless you name it. To see and notice the feelings requires us to develop our own skills of mindfulness. Dr Ronald Epstein at the University of Rochester has taught mindfulness training for health care professionals for years. He describes and documents the multiple benefits—both for patients and providers—in his excellent book *Attending*.[10]

THE OTHER EMOTION(S)

In medical school, there is about as much education on emotions as on nutrition. It's paltry. Who decided these topics were unimportant? Trained as we are in a stagnant system, we physicians stand to learn a lot from other team members when it comes to both emotions and nutrition. In the realm of feelings, fear can masquerade as a lot of different emotions and affects, including apprehensive, concerned, dread, angry, hesitant, mistrustful, panicked, petrified, reserved, scared, sensitive, shaky, suspicious, terrified, timid, trepidation, unnerved, wary, worried, and unsteady. Realize (or remember) that as we first meet people feeling these feelings, we're also asking them to consider life-altering decisions in this mental space. Feelings wax and wane. Being prepared to address them whenever they arise is part of whole person care.

Bringing books and training materials into staff development meetings is a good way to bring these topics up for discussion and learning. Figure 7.1 shows an adaptation of one such tool demonstrating how feeling states like fear and vulnerability can transition to more tolerable states when needs are met. Most staff are grateful for the opportunity to talk about the daily elephants in the room.

When needs ARE NOT being met		When needs ARE being met	
Fearful		**Curious**	
• Apprehensive	• Suspicious	• Adventurous	• Inquisitive
• Concerned	• Terrified	• Alert	• Fascinated
• Dread	• Timid	• Interested	• Spellbound
• Fearful	• Trepidation	• Intrigued	• Stimulated
• Foreboding	• Unnerved		
• Frightened	• Wary		
• Hesitant	• Worried		
• Mistrustful	• Reserved		
• Panicked	• Sensitive		
• Petrified	• Shaky		
• Scared	• Unsteady		
Vulnerable		**Confident**	
• Cautious	• Insecure	• Empowered	• Secure
• Fragile	• Leery	• Proud	• Self Assured
• Guarded	• Reluctant	• Safe	
• Helpless			

Figure 7.1 How Needs Impact Feelings

Example of how feeling states can transmute based on needs, as adapted from the Center for School Transformation, Compassionate Communication. On the left side are the emotions that happen when our needs are not met—emotions that contract and restrict. On the right side are emotions when our needs are met—emotions that relax and open. Jampolsky called these "fear" and "love."

Another view is shared by Gerald Jampolsky, MD, in his book *Love is Letting Go of Fear*.[11] A short, impactful read full of cartoons (in case someone on your team doesn't read anything but medical journals), it's now in its third edition, with over 4 million copies sold. Dr Jampolsky taught there are only two emotions: love and fear, and they are opposites. As a medical student, Dr Jonas was so intrigued and confused by this book that he went to visit Dr Jampolsky to ask for his help in understanding it. He recalls:

> Before the meeting I had always thought that hate was the opposite of love. Dr Jampolsky corrected me. Hate, he said, is just another manifestation of fear. Both hate and fear tighten a person and narrow their view, making it more likely they will not see the truth. Love, on the other hand, loosens our narrow views and opens our mind. In my experience, this allows us to see more of reality than we would otherwise, to see the whole picture, and so care for the whole person. From this position we can make better decisions. And we often feel better.

Cancer care is done out of love. It's why you have made it this far in the book, despite having a million other things to do. Our challenge is to hold that space, day-to-day, as an antidote to fear.

WHO'S THE BOSS?

At diagnosis, when patients are immediately vulnerable and relying on us for direction, we find ourselves considering how much ownership is really of interest to the person at this delicate time? How much can we expect them to decide for themselves while they are also dealing with information overload and fear? Do we just hand down the standard of care treatment plan? Or do we take some time to learn more about what matters more to the person: length or quality of life? Does the person want just the broad overview and schedule information, barely considering the drug information sheets we've dutifully provided? Or are they the kind of person who wants to hear a granular level of detail within the consent process? It depends and it can change.

"First do no harm" is a dance we may do differently with different people. We do it best if we find out about the person up front and learn what makes them unique from all the patients we have cared for before. If we don't do this, we are more likely to misstep, make possibly false assumptions, and start down the treatment road unaligned.

Dr McManamon likes to tell patients preparing for treatment, "You're the boss. If you say stop, we stop. If you have a question, we answer. It's our job to worry about all the what ifs of treatment, to worry enough to keep you safe, but it's your job to tell us the truth of what you are experiencing and want in our care." For example, when patients start on an oxaliplatin-based therapy, after counseling about potential side effects, Dr McManamon sometimes shares this story:

> During my fellowship training in DC, I treated a young FBI agent diagnosed with colon cancer. Like you, after surgery he was starting chemotherapy containing the drug oxaliplatin, the one that can cause the cold sensitivity I've told you about. In those days we gave oxaliplatin for 6 months straight, more than we do now because we now know more is not better. He came in every 2 weeks for chemo and always said everything was fine. He worked the whole time. He always came alone and was very focused on completing the course of therapy. Then one day he came in shuffling, admitting he was suffering with electrical shock-like pains in his legs. We put him on an immediate work restriction, saying "No gun carry." He then told us he had been hiding progressive symptoms for weeks because he wanted to complete the full planned course of treatment. Please don't suffer in silence. Let us know if you have any symptoms of concern, even if we don't ask. But when we do ask, we need you to tell us the honest truth. Remember, you're the boss.

WHEN THEY COME ALONE

At diagnosis, it quickly becomes apparent who is going to have more trouble getting through treatment. It's the people who come alone. Delving deeper within a first visit to oncology, when the team learns a person newly diagnosed with cancer has no one who could accompany them today, there's a shared heartbreak. At the VA, Dr McManamon has been shocked at how many veterans "do cancer" alone.

The US Surgeon General's report on loneliness cites our workplaces as a cause, but many people are no longer in the workforce and yet are alone. Wherever it starts, we see the effects of loneliness and isolation daily in cancer care. When we take someone's vital signs, shake their hand that first visit, or examine for a vein or heart sounds, we may be the only one who has touched this person in years. It is a sacred understanding from which to provide whole person cancer care. We know from both scientific data collected and observation that people facing cancer alone don't typically do as well. Maybe when they come alone, we need to find out why and, if needed, begin an amped-up care plan and get the social worker involved from the first visit. Maybe when they come alone, we need to ask more about what they need, right away. The questions on the Personal Health Inventory screen patients for social and emotional needs, so we know we should address these and loneliness in whole person care. But most of us don't need a special screening tool to see and feel loneliness.

In cases where there's no support network, a call to the primary care physician or referring provider may create a safety net around the person. Do everything you can when they come alone—this is an all-hands-on-deck situation. If your clinic can't imagine a workflow where every patient gets a HOPE visit, at least consider patients who can't identify a potential caregiver in an emergency as a place to start.

The solution to loneliness is a true friend, someone who has your back and will both call you on your responsibility and support you through your weaknesses and needs. We discuss formal means

THE DFCI NEW DIAGNOSIS BUNDLE

1. Understand the patient medically and personally, including cultural beliefs, decision-making style, family support, living conditions, and financial situation.

2. Create a structured treatment plan that is informed by multidisciplinary participants and a patient's unique needs, which summarizes pertinent test results and a course of action, and that is accessible to both patients and providers.

3. Time educational efforts appropriately, by incorporating input from the patient and the family about what they want to know and their level of comprehension.

4. Help the patient and family maintain control over their lives and manage their emotional reactions.

5. Minimize anxiety related to needless waiting for information or next steps.

of social support in Chapter 2. One meta-analysis of more than 80 studies showed that social support decreased the risk of mortality from 12 to 25%, depending on the type of support.[12] In cancer care, shared spaces such as waiting and infusion rooms should be designed to be both safe and conducive to social interactions.

We can't talk about loneliness without reflecting on the COVID-19 times we've lived through. In oncology, the effects were well-documented. We were able to stay afloat with virtual visits, where at least we could see each other's faces (often for the first time). Digital social support, while not as good as person-to-person contact, is still better that no contact.[13]

Well before the pandemic, evidence showed that loneliness and social isolation endanger human health, in part by inducing stress. And chronic stress can induce tumorigenesis and promote cancer development.[14] Waiting for a cancer diagnosis is as stressful as it gets. For people diagnosed during the pandemic, there was more waiting than usual, compounded by supply chain issues and workforce shortages. More and more, areas of alignment across cancer care institutions strive to support the whole person and their caregivers, in the time of diagnosis and beyond. The Dana-Farber Cancer Institute (DFCI) has suggested a 10-day window for a "new diagnosis bundle" of specific, person-centered care following diagnosis. As your team considers how or where to make whole person cancer care occur in a day's workflow, it may be helpful to consider the 5 foundational principles DFCI identified as most impactful for people around the time of initial diagnosis. The principles give your team a reference point for assessing any whole person cancer care pilot programs you may be considering.[15]

Consider with your team where you already meet many of these principles and how you could succeed in meeting more of them or meeting them more completely.

DISPARITIES IN DIAGNOSIS

In the US, we know that zip code matters when it comes to health and longevity. For example, research has shown that information on race at a zip code level is associated both with less preventive care, such as colorectal cancer screening, and rates of higher stage at diagnosis.[16,17] Access to health care (and insurance) and factors such as the "social deprivation index" or SDI play a large part in whether screening occurs, and have downstream effects in mortality.

Numerous documented examples of disparities in diagnosis exist due to racism, socioeconomic status, age, geography, language, sex, disability, citizenship status, and sexual identity (gender) and orientation. Knowing that our system (and us in it) cares for and treats certain populations inadequately is a first step for teams to create processes to help correct these disparities. Active consideration of social determinants of health by teams helps people get the care they need at diagnosis and beyond.[18] Disparities exist during all phases of the cancer journey, so awareness of and dealing with the drivers of disparities at diagnosis, treatment (see Chapter 8), and after treatment (see Chapters 9 and 10) is needed. Many of the approaches and tools we describe in this book, such as peer partners, patient advocates, group visits, and empowerment methods, have application with these populations, especially if used from the time of first diagnosis.

A FIRST STEP

As you and your team adopt whole person care tools and create new ones, consider how they can be used from the time of diagnosis. Be aware of how people newly diagnosed can make only so much progress on their own, especially the ones who have no one outside of our team to turn to.

At the Dayton VA Medical Center, an oncology nurse navigator identified that veterans and their caregivers were stressed by possibly unrealistic expectations of how fast things should or could occur following a diagnosis. With others she began a "Pathways to Treatment" group class that specifically introduced information on expected timelines to treatment (for example, turnaround of additional testing such as next-generation sequencing following biopsy, or for steps required before the first fraction of radiation). The idea for Pathways to Treatment began when the navigator became aware of veterans' suffering. This awareness grew into a joint effort with the radiation nurse navigator, and others from departments like nutrition and mental health. At the class, veterans and caregivers have time to share concerns and anxieties, while also meeting each other and building community from the time of diagnosis. Pathways to Treatment, like DCFI's new patient care bundle, tries to address the suffering that can follow diagnosis. It's a good first step.

SUMMARY POINTS

- Fear follows the word cancer—testing repeats fear, waiting for information increases it.

- Know the patient—does the team hold more fear than this patient at diagnosis?

- Create a safe environment—physically and emotionally—an optimal healing environment.

- Name possible emotions and make space for them (by listening).

- Learn how not to misuse prognostic data to increase fear and produce a nocebo effect.

- Address provider burnout and poor communication skills—these can be improved.

- Pay special attention to someone alone or subject to racial or other drivers of disparities.

- Improve, streamline, and standardize patient care delivery at the time of cancer diagnosis.

CHAPTER EIGHT

TREATMENT

As research progresses, people with cancer face a greater number of treatment choices and the need to balance an ever-broadening range of off-target effects. Care teams involved in cancer treatment planning must shepherd people through increasingly complex choice paradigms.

Whether a cancer diagnosis adds to a long list of preexisting conditions or not, some people have high medical literacy and others do not. Gauging that level and where to begin a conversation on treatment options is one of the most valuable skills teams can hone. Which treatment options are offered as optimal comes from teams' knowledge base, a grounding in the standard of care in practice, time learning about new research findings, and an ability to reach out to colleagues with additional expertise or experience when necessary. As new approaches and knowledge arise at lightening pace, it is hard to keep up and align the science, the practice, and the person. People come to the treatment discussion expecting answers and hope. In this chapter, we will look at whole person care within the realm of treatment goals, choice, and timing.

THE GOALS OF CANCER TREATMENT

One of the most important issues for determining the value of a treatment are the goals desired and outcomes sought and measured. Those goals may be multiple, and may conflict, requiring a delicate balance. Jan needed to juggle at least 5 different goals when deciding how to treat her cancers. Length of survival was important, as was the presence or absence of the cancer. These goals were what her oncologists emphasized. But, over the years, these goals weren't the only ones and often, not the most important ones to her. The ability to live the type of life she wanted—working, caring for kids and grandkids, traveling, spending time with friends and family—were also key. How she felt physically was also important. Was she going to feel sick, have pain, be tired all the time, not be able to hear, feel her feet, or think during or after the treatment? Finally, she wanted (as we all do) to have hope and confidence in the decisions made. If she left an appointment without all these goals discussed, even if they conflicted with each other, that confidence and hope was difficult to achieve.

Figure 8.1 illustrates Jan's cancer care world when she got breast cancer. On the right-hand side is what the oncology team brought to her and was trying to implement. Most of it focused on diagnosis and treatment of the tumor, although from Jan's perspective the stage 1 tumor had been removed by surgery. On the left-hand side are some of the other things Jan was concerned about in the management of her cancer. These were the priorities in her life—that is, what mattered to her. Time to help care for her young children was paramount.

This situation involves information overload for everyone. Her oncologist knew practically nothing about what was on the left-hand side, although the cancer nurses would often talk to her about them and ask how they were going, sometimes working to coordinate her treatments to accommodate those goals. No formal support for discussing these areas was ever mentioned by the oncology team. Jan discovered accidentally that there was an entire center affiliated with the hospital available to support the

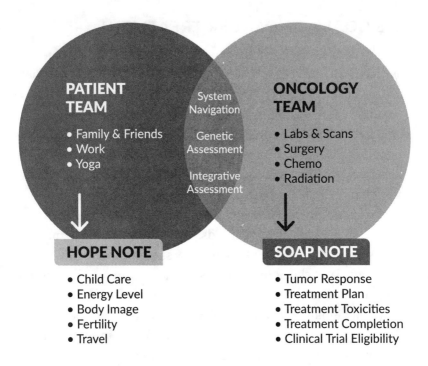

Figure 8.1 The Person's World and the Provider's World

On the left side are the issues Jan was concerned about as her treatment plan evolved. On the right side was what her oncology team was focused on. Goals are somewhat different. Information overload is the same.

left-hand side of her world through free to low-cost services like counseling, social work, nutrition, exercise, yoga, acupuncture, support groups, spiritual services, and art therapy. And so, without the help of her cancer care team and unbeknownst to them, Jan began to engage in those services. To the hospital's credit, many of these services were later picked up and made available on site—eventually becoming prominently featured in their diagnostic and infusion centers. Whole person care was emerging at the hospital.

When determining the best treatment plan for a patient, the whole team must weigh not only what they will do but the value of that doing compared to alternatives including doing nothing or less. In appropriate cases, even when "doing nothing" for the cancer, there is opportunity to help patients improve aspects of their health and wellbeing.

"DOING NOTHING": AN OPPORTUNITY FOR HEALTH PROMOTION

While treatment overload is often the problem, no treatment may also present a challenge, yet is sometimes appropriate, for example in diagnoses not requiring next steps of surgery, radiation, or targeted oral and intravenous therapies. For observation as treatment course, patient education and support is standard, but of a lesser intensity. For low-risk chronic lymphocytic leukemia (CLL) or low-risk prostate cancer (PC), following discussion of prognosis we offer a follow up and lab monitoring schedule. Although straightforward, the person embarks on a path of anticipation or anxiety, depending on how well their needs for information and reassurance have been met. "Doing nothing" is in effect what a person with low-risk CLL or PC may hear when we suggest observation and tracking of blood labs and can be a lead into all manner of patient responses, from undisclosed exploration of alternative therapies to dramatic lifestyle change considerations on their part. If the information on observation as treatment plan resonates as intended, the person's listening can shift from "doing nothing" to an opportunity for whole person care and a reorientation to activities that will help prevent chronic illness in general and enhance wellbeing as discussed in Chapter 4.

At the first visit during an agreed upon period of observation, we can ask about what matters to the person and about what ways they have been strengthening their wellbeing since we last met. We can help them focus on what may be their real risks (such as heart disease) and help them mitigate those risks and support their health and functioning. Visits during observation may be some of the most teachable moments for all of us. Observation doesn't have to mean "doing nothing," it can be a health-promoting period and a chance for our teams to strengthen a role as supportive healers in an otherwise low-risk episode of care.

A patient of Dr Jonas shows how this can happen. Frank was 64 and had rising PSA tests found during his annual physical. A prostate biopsy found low-risk cancer. He also had prediabetes, high LDL cholesterol and a high cardiac calcium score with a family history of early death from heart disease. He elected to "watch and wait" on his prostate cancer but embarked on improving his diet (Mediterranean) and regular exercise, statins, metformin and genistein supplements. Off target effects were some welcome weight loss and increased energy. Two years later his PSA was normal and a repeat prostate biopsy found no evidence of cancer. Equally important was that his cardiac risk had markedly improved with low LDL cholesterol, normal hemoglobin A1C and, remarkably, a lower cardiac calcium score. In his case, the diagnosis of cancer helped him get healthier all around.

WHOLE PERSON TREATMENT PLANS

Unfortunately, most patients with cancer require more than observation. In those situations, our first step is to create a treatment plan that takes advantage of all we know to offer. The key is continuing to expand on "all we know" to transition from a conventional oncology care plan to a more whole person cancer care plan. While both require use of standard approved therapies, they tend to look different. Here's why (and some examples).

CaLM and Home

What do the words "calm" and "home" bring to mind? Safety? Relaxation? For many they suggest an idealized way of care. When used in relation to cancer treatment, they invoke something beyond the slash and burn of killing cells. If you participate in an oncology medical home model, you may see examples of how the word home embodies and reinforces certain aspects of caring.

In the CaLM Model, CaLM stands for Cancer Life ReiMagined and is a model anchored in the oncology medical home (OMH) and collaborative care approaches.[1] Piloted at the Livestrong® Cancer Institutes at University of Texas Health Austin, the CaLM

Model of Whole-Person Cancer Care™ "set out to build a model that treats the mind, body, and heart, as one entity."

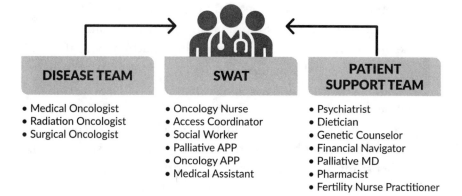

DISEASE TEAM
- Medical Oncologist
- Radiation Oncologist
- Surgical Oncologist

SWAT
- Oncology Nurse
- Access Coordinator
- Social Worker
- Palliative APP
- Oncology APP
- Medical Assistant

PATIENT SUPPORT TEAM
- Psychiatrist
- Dietician
- Genetic Counselor
- Financial Navigator
- Palliative MD
- Pharmacist
- Fertility Nurse Practitioner

Figure 8.2 The CaLM Staffing Model of Whole Person Cancer Care

On the left is the cancer treatment team. On the right is the person support team. In the middle are those on the team-focused integration of these groups for whole person care. Reprinted with permission from the Association of Community Cancer Centers. Original figure from: Schear RM, Eckhardt SG, Richardson R, Jones B, Kvale E. Cancer Life reiMagined: The CaLM Model of Whole Person Cancer Care. Oncol Issues. 2020;35(4):22-35.

The program won the 2019 Association of Community Cancer Centers' Innovator Award. Interestingly, CaLM's paradigm still includes kill-related terminology, the so-called "SWAT Team" which is the primary team. But CaLM places this team within the oncology medical home responsible for a person's care and includes an oncology advanced practice provider, supportive care and survivorship doctor, oncology social worker, nurse navigator, medical assistant, and community navigator. In the CaLM model, oncology physicians, medical, radiation and surgical, are on "the disease team" and do not see the patient every visit. If this model looks of interest, consider how you and your team could tap into the aspects that your patients may resonate with to provide whole person care.

DOING LESS

Oncology today is moving toward doing less. Examples include the minimally invasive procedures, liquid biopsies, lessened chemotherapy and radiation. Other examples include clinical trials such as the French Stop Imatinib study in chronic myeloid leukemia (CML).[2] This study showed that imatinib can safely be discontinued in patients with the blood cancer CML who have had undetectable minimal residual disease for at least 2 years on treatment if certain baseline criteria are also met. It is probably not a coincidence that the French, practicing in cost-conscious system of universal health care, were the first to do such a trial. Another study was done in Japan, also with a system of universal health care.[3] Such investigations are about quality of life, financial savings, and choice; they're less about profits, one size fits all, and cancer eradication at any cost. In the French study, investigators found that if a patient met the criteria to stop imatinib and the disease returned, the person was just as likely to go back into remission with resumption of therapy as they had been at initial therapy. When an approach shifts polarity toward doing less, we lead into a whole person cancer care model. Less toxicity, more quality of life, lower overall costs.

Less surgery is also being tested, especially in certain cancers known to have early metastasis. In pancreatic cancer, a study of Minimally Invasive Pancreatic Surgery (MIPS) was compared to usual more extensive and aggressive, so called "open," surgery or Open Pancreatic Surgery (OPS). MIPS produced longer disease free and overall life expectancy and fewer side effects than OPS. The study involved 396 patients. The median overall and disease-free survival after MIPS was 30.7 months and 14.8 months, respectively, versus 20.3 months and 10.7 months, respectively, compared to OPS.[4]

Deescalating therapy is a long-coming and welcome trend. Radiation, a technology-heavy paradigm, continues to evolve to allow shorter course treatments, such as single fraction gamma knife for appropriate brain or other tumors, stereotactic body radiotherapy

(SBRT), given in 3 to 5 fractions for lung or other tumors, and abbreviated courses of radiation for small cell lung cancers.

When certain criteria are met, we can leave postlumpectomy radiation out of a treatment plan entirely. Jan got the full 33 sessions for the first breast cancer when she was young. When 25 years later in age, recently published data shows that omission of postoperative radiation applies to women over 65 with ER-positive breast cancers meeting certain criteria.[5]

Dr McManamon learned how to do less from a memorable patient:

> I first met my patient with left-side ER-positive breast cancer in the postlumpectomy setting. To complete the 28-33 sessions of Monday through Friday radiation that was most common then, in 2009, was, she had said, out of the question because she worked. She wanted to avoid any cosmetic effects she could from exposing the whole breast and protect her heart. I nearly poo-pooed her suggestion of radioactive seeds inserted through a catheter to be placed in the breast tumor cavity because the 5-day regime seemed too good to be true.
>
> Although I encouraged her to discuss with her radiation oncologist, a loose read of our interaction would suggest I brushed her off. Looking back, I can see that a call to a radiation colleague would have been useful here, or at least some human curiosity on my part, but in a busy clinic and starting to find my way just out of training, all I gave her was a lecture about the standard. It's an example of my hubris and, from what I could tell, her frustration. Due to her persistence and self-advocacy, we continued within a therapeutic relationship that included standard hormonal therapy following her completion of the 5-day radiation schedule.

The more closed we are to seeing what it is we don't know (which is always going to be a lot) or the higher the stakes we perceive when it comes to something we don't know about (for example, someone having an "unnecessarily bad outcome"), the greater the chance to miss what is most appropriate to a person's care. If we fast-forward from 2009, multiple studies now support use of partial breast irradiation in low-risk early breast cancer.[6]

In whole person cancer care, we each consider what it would be like to undergo treatment and make changes in our care accordingly. This requires more than release of hubris. It involves ever increasing empathy, less othering and more asking ourselves, "What if it was me?" By working as a team to find strength in our differences, learning together what we don't now know, we make things better for all people facing cancer.

EARLY WHOLE PERSON TREATMENT PLANNING

There is a need for whole person care planning at the beginning of treatment planning. We see the consequences of not doing that regularly. The following quotes, both from recent patients, should not be entirely surprising. From a woman with breast cancer living in a rural area: "I guess you could say I went into this kind of blindly. I didn't ask enough questions. I found out by chance about reconstruction. I didn't know if I could afford it. No one around me ever talked about it."[7] From a man with rectal cancer: "However, although my life has been spared, the quality of that life is gone, perhaps forever...At the very least, I should have been offered referrals to sexual health specialists and support groups, so I could have gotten help sooner. A few years after the surgery... I became so depressed about my situation that I called the suicide hotline. I don't think I was seriously considering taking my own life, but the thought frightened me enough to seek counseling with a sexual health therapist."[8]

These 2 people describe their recent experience of treatment in ways that we may find shocking. Teams strive to do a great job, and most would say we do a good job, but how can this be true when people are still having such experiences? To find out where your care may sit in terms of these needs, consider asking patients who have been through the system where you work. Those kinds of surveys can provide important data and guidance on how to improve care where you work and serve as a basis for practice improvement.

Racism as a Barrier to Treatment Outcome

In Chapter 7 we discussed how racism and other drivers of disparities in care influence diagnosis. These factors operate during treatment also. When we look at the factors known to generate health, we can see how disease-causing factors are more present when core wellness factors are absent. Race and poverty are structural drivers for much of this absence.

Besides lower rates of cancer screening in certain minority populations as a means of prevention, multiple disparities occur between different populations and subgroups in cancer treatment and outcomes. In the 2022 cancer statistics for American Indian and Alaska Native (AIAN) individuals, overall cancer rates among AIAN individuals were 2% higher than among white individuals for incidence (2014 through 2018, confined to Purchased/Referred Care Delivery Area counties to reduce racial misclassification) but 18% higher for mortality (2015 through 2019). A well-designed observational study published in 2020 found that among patients treated in VA health care system—where all patients have equal access to care—African American men did not appear to have more-aggressive prostate cancer at the time of diagnosis or a higher death rate from the disease than non-Hispanic white men.[9] Of course, retrospective data like this does not show causation (i.e., equal access to care may not be the only factor at play in the findings showing lack of racial disparity). Evaluating and addressing how racism and other disparity drivers may operate in your system and can be corrected is an important additional opportunity to improve quality of care.

USUAL CARE? NO ONE IS AVERAGE

For any cancer diagnosis requiring treatment, people are offered treatment modalities and consultations with providers who can hopefully explain the risk versus benefit scenario. If there is an agreement to accept treatment, information on side effects is provided by informed consent to allow it to get started. Often there's a feeling of urgency to get through these steps quickly, regardless of the nature of the tumor's actual biology, particularly if this aspect is unknown. The urgency is also simply human nature: don't just sit there, do something. The rush acts as counterweight to any uncertainty the patient and team may experience. But in the haste to get started, the full menu of options may not be considered. At this point, the most common options present the path of least resistance; the person with cancer gravitates to the clinician who seems most confident.

To be sure, in some cancers, the rush is required. For a 60-year-old woman with metastatic ampullary adenocarcinoma, the goal was to get treatment started as soon as possible, in support of her wish for prolongation of life and amelioration of cancer-associated pain. She underwent germline testing (no variant to target). A celiac plexus block did not provide relief. She embarked on chemotherapy with the hope it would decrease her pain and was seen by the palliative care service. Expected side effects began and were initially tolerated; when they became increasingly and unexpectedly severe, she was readmitted within the first cycle. Only in retrospect does the team fully understand the risks and benefits of treatment, rather than palliative care alone. All involved quickly see that some of the assumptions of risk versus benefit were erroneous. She is now living through the consequences.

When a new treatment is approved (with its requisite Kaplan-Meier progression free or overall survival curve), it is usually accompanied by an analysis of side effects and explanation that they are "tolerable," based on toxicity grading scales used in clinical research. Even with standardized ways of measuring side effects (for example, CTCAE Grades 1-5, with 5 being death), we know that tolerability can only be in the eye of the individual patient. Who decides (and how) whether a sequence of 33 radiation sessions, or 6, 3-drug chemotherapy cycles, is tolerable? Is a 7 or a 10% increase in 5-year life expectancy worth the risk of preventing a patient from doing what matters most in life? Those are a lot of variables for a patient to weigh. Yet, it *is* up to the patient, whether they understand or not.

When Jan started treatment for her ovarian cancer the first time, she stuck closely to the schedule. She was too tired to care for grandchildren and to do community work. The second time around, she realized that the timing of treatment could be modified to still get in everything her oncologist wanted while allowing her to do more of the activities she valued. She varied the cycle of treatment and closely followed the response to be sure it was working. As her fatigue got progressively worse and the fifth cycle approached, her oncologist suggested that she might try fasting for 24 to 48 hours before chemotherapy to see if that might blunt the side effects.[10]

PERSONALIZED CARE AND SIDE EFFECTS

In some practices doing more whole person care with personalized care plans is prioritized to address patient specific side effects. Before treatment starts and armed with the list of potential side effects from the informed consent process, the care team asks what from the list most concerns the patient. An advocate, family member or not, is present for this discussion. From there, that most concerning item is addressed. For Jan, it was time toxicity, not concern for the direct side effects of chemotherapy. For another, it might be a needle phobia. Or hair loss. Neuropathy, brain fog, or weight gain or loss. The care team then takes time to address the most concerning issue or highest stake potential side effect up front, even before treatment starts.

During this time, communication about the likelihood of these effects and ways to mitigate them can blunt the nocebo problems that might be induced by the usual informed consent process we discussed in Chapter 6—simply reading the list of potential effects. Considerable research shows that simply telling a patient about potential side effects of a treatment increases the likelihood of getting them.[11] This presents an ethical dilemma. Accurate information needs to be conveyed to the patient. However, the usual way a clinician or pharmacist does this (by reading the list of side effects without framing or context) has potential to harm the patient. Time spent to understand how a patient receives, believes, and processes this information can mitigate and help reduce these harms. Some patients shrug the list off. Some take it to heart and start looking for symptoms after the first dose. Unfortunately, few pharmacists or clinicians are trained in how to properly communicate side effects in a manner that blunts the nocebo effect by specifying which are rare, which are mild, and how average probability data does not mean the patient will get the side effect.[12]

For example, if a person is most concerned with neuropathy because it could impact their quality of life as a musician, modalities to decrease the risk, such as cooling extremities during chemotherapy infusion, or acupuncture, would be set up. During treatment, infusion room nurses are empowered to speak up on the person's behalf if any concerns are raised and they can do so because the standard has been elevated and agreed upon: providing whole person care. It is known that, in this clinic, we do better than just tolerate expected side effects. It may even be a poster on the wall of the treatment room, inviting people to speak up, or an actual invitation to each patient to consider how a patient advocate could benefit them along the treatment journey and a list of supportive options and their availability.

If a person does not know what a patient advocate does, they could be informed through a video clip shared directly, or in a variety of ways. The main message is that we as a team invite the person to choose an advocate to represent their best interests. That person may be the patient (some can do this), a family member or friend, a formal or hired advocate, or a member of the care team itself. It need not be the institution's advocate. Before treatment starts, for those who identify they want to actively explore ways to feel better during and after treatment, it may mean a Healing-Oriented Practices and Environments (HOPE) visit to find out what that looks like for the person, what areas of health they wish to strengthen going into treatment and beyond. In our experience, a HOPE visit helps patients voice concerns they have about their own health practices and is a person-driven discussion of where they may wish to make change, however incremental.

YOU ALREADY KNOW HOW TO DO WHOLE PERSON CARE

If you've never (until reading this book) heard of the Personal Health Inventory (PHI) as a tool or the HOPE visit as a possibility, we suspect that you still already provide many aspects of whole person care at the time of new diagnoses and during treatment. We guess you also do it outside of your usual job environment. If you have any connection to cancer care, you are seen as a conduit to valuable information, a trusted source.

As Dr McManamon says:

> I'm at the age where my high school friends and their parents are facing new cancer diagnoses. They call me to get an initial understanding of the prognosis, treatment paradigms, what to expect from treatment, and what they can do to get through it. When I have a conversation with the father of one of these dear friends, I already know who they are— I've been in their homes, their cars, at their kitchen tables, and in their now-adult children's lives for decades. It's a special place from which to provide *pro bono* consultation. Some of the most rewarding interactions I've had as a healer started from a place of well-rounded understanding and trust built over years—and from an all-in emotional investment.

Each of you reading this knows inherently how to provide whole person cancer care. Whatever role you play on your care team, if you work in oncology in any capacity, someone has reached out personally to you for guidance. And you've met the calls with grace and generosity. You've connected them to the right resources. If this doesn't resonate for you personally, consider why. It could be a sign of burnout and needs not being met.

PACE AND PAUSING

Some diagnoses require immediate moves to treatment; others allow more time for decision-making. Research in this area suggests that in some cases, we have more time for treatment planning than our internal urgency may suggest. In breast cancer, the increasing use of neoadjuvant chemotherapy when indicated means that the time to surgery is lengthening. If surgery is instead the first modality following diagnosis, scheduling the procedure by 90 days, should the person need that much time, can be acceptable.[13] For best outcomes in muscle-invasive bladder cancer, similar scenarios would include surgery within 24 weeks after neoadjuvant chemotherapy or within 90 days if they didn't receive up-front chemotherapy.[14,15]

For cancers with accurate markers of cancer growth, treatment and timing can be more carefully individualized. Someday, liquid biopsy and blood monitoring may make this universal. Teams can provide the voice of reason when it comes to treatment timing. Care planning is possibly our biggest role within advocacy for whole person cancer care. Our teams are aware of data on time to treatment and toxicity, so they are equipped to assist people in the throes of fear following diagnosis. Allowing for a pause in planning can make a difference. When the person with cancer and the family have a say and are fully aligned with the plan, even if it is in small variables of timing, they are more empowered to speak up along the journey.

THE INTERNET AS ADVOCATE OR ENEMY

All people, patients, and providers alike, explore complementary and alternative care options via the internet. As they do, they encounter social media influencers on platforms such as Instagram—which means they encounter people who tout magic devices or special concoctions with ingredients you've never heard of, conveniently linked in their bio for purchase. Most patients can ignore what they find online, but it's typical that friends and family members pile on with "helpful" suggestions that are heavy on anecdote and search engine input. Some of the approaches that emerge from these information streams may be helpful. Some may be safe but not proven. Some may be bolstered by substantial evidence but aren't yet reimbursed by insurance. And some may be dangerous. The increase in AI will likely make facts even more difficult to find online.

Part of our job as care teams is to understand the pressure people are under when it comes to treatment decisions. We're not the only ones telling them what to do. Revisit the Four Ps model introduced in Chapter 6 for ways to help us help people with cancer navigate the advocacy of the internet and well-meaning others. And in Chapter 2, a patient and advocate provide both her story and guidelines for using online resources, social media, and chat rooms.

WHEN AN ADVOCATE OVERSTEPS

If you've been in oncology practice long enough to see the ebb and flow of health trends, which means really anyone reading this, you have seen much change. One day we hear of the benefits of the ketogenic diet[16] and the next we hear it's best to fast, such as with Dr Valter Longo's fasting mimicking diet.[17]

One of our colleagues cared for a woman with glioblastoma multiforme (GBM), a near-uniformly fatal brain tumor. Based on some suggestive research, she and her husband decided she would follow a ketogenic diet. On this, combined with conventional treatment, the tumor was shrinking, but so was she. Over time, with stable disease, she was less enthusiastic about the diet, but was bolstered by her spouse's zeal for ketosis. When they came to appointments, she was thin, weak, and sarcopenic; he brought a spreadsheet of her "in-range" blood sugar trends. She reported missing foods not on the diet plan and wanted a break. He was certain that the diet was working because the tumor wasn't growing.

The choice to go on the ketogenic diet was fully within her scope of self-directed treatment and based on data. But when dietary restrictions became stifling and the patient was clearly unhappy with them, it was time for the team to embody the role of protector, if only to give supportive voice to her concerns and her quality of life. In fact, there was a tension related to this dietary intervention as promoted by her caregiver, with the team and her husband increasingly at odds. Partnership was difficult to navigate but the nature of this guiding principle allowed the care team to support her wishes even through a period of contention with her caregiver. In the end, she did relax her dietary intake and sometime later succumbed to the disease. She lived years above the usual expectation for GBM, perhaps because of the ketogenic diet—and perhaps despite it.

When we promote treatment interventions, we look to balance protection of the whole person in a true partnership. In oncology, we have chosen a field where we step past the tenet of "First, do no harm" to get to something greater, whether that be disease control, cure or allowing any person's stated goal in life to be met. Even in observation as treatment, there is a potential degree of harm we navigate together. What makes this paradox of treatment bearable is that it occurs within a relationship. As the late bell hooks wrote, "rarely, if ever, are any of us healed in isolation. Healing is an act of communion."[18]

That's part of how healing works in cancer treatment. Let's move now to see how healing can continue to be supported in the period following active treatment.

SUMMARY POINTS

- Navigating treatment is complex and usually results in information overload for everyone involved.

- Understanding patients' goals early on can help develop a better treatment plan.

- Models such as Cancer Life ReiMagined (CaLM) are examples of whole person care in practice.

- Doing less and de-escalation is gaining traction in oncology as a guiding principle.

- Racism, sexism, and agism biases built into treatment culture, can be noticed and addressed.

- Alignment of "what matters" to the person with treatment risk and benefit is of paramount importance in planning.

CHAPTER NINE

AFTER TREATMENT

When someone with cancer completes treatment, one long, arduous leg of their cancer journey is done. For some, adjuvant or maintenance therapy continues, possibly over years. Regardless of therapy continuation or not, the need for whole person care also remains.[1] With completion of any part of a treatment journey, there is a pause of sorts. This has been described by many people as the other hardest part—the after treatment, when the so-called "new normal" of life can surprise in ways both pleasant and not. Most of us on cancer care teams recognize this period as survivorship.

According to the NCI, "An individual is considered a cancer survivor from the time of diagnosis through the balance of life. There are many types of survivors, including those living with cancer and those free of cancer. This term is meant to capture a population of those with a history of cancer rather than to provide a label that may or may not resonate with individuals."

We use the word survivor here for convenience, but no one wants to simply survive without the presence of wellbeing or promise of hope. We encourage those of you who work with patients to ask what terms fit best when you design programs around survivorship. Some ideas include "wellness after cancer," "optimal recovery," or "thrivorship." However, only your patients can tell you what they care to be called—maybe just by their name. No one likes to be labeled. By asking your patients, you are very likely to learn something.

Survivorship is often seen as the third phase in the cancer journey, one that involves health maintenance and prevention of recurrence. Outside of the few places with well-staffed and robust survivorship clinics, overall, we don't do it very well. Conventional cancer clinics that provide a survivorship care plan, following Commission on Cancer and other directives, struggle to do so. Most often, they provide plans only in cases where they're required. In this chapter we describe ways in which to improve the survivorship phase through a whole person perspective and care approach.

SURVIVOR STATISTICS

Better early cancer detection and treatment mean that today many people with cancer are living years beyond diagnosis and treatment. As of January 2022, there were an estimated 18.1 million cancer survivors in the US—approximately 5.4% of the country's population. The number of cancer survivors is projected to increase by 24.4%, to 22.5 million, by 2032. By 2040, that number is projected to grow to 26.0 million.

In 2022, 69% of survivors have lived 5 years or more since their diagnosis; 47% of survivors have lived 10 years or more since their diagnosis; and 18% of survivors have lived 20 years or more.[2]

In the US, about 624,000 people are living with the most common metastatic cancers (breast, prostate, lung, colorectal, bladder cancer, or metastatic melanoma). By 2025, that number is expected to increase to about 694,000.[3] All of these numbers represent our work and service, as well as the strength and resolve of patients and caregivers to make it through treatment and beyond.

However, people living with a history of cancer may experience a range of ongoing challenges in every dimension, starting with quality of life. Some 37% of adult survivors say they have some difficulty with basic activities of daily living, while 55% report being unable to live independently.[4] Among older people with a history of cancer, 64% say they have functional limitations that affect their mobility or activities of daily living.[5]

Basic prevention and core wellness and lifestyle factors have the greatest impact on long-term survival and quality of life for people with cancer, just as they do for those without it. In addition to supporting the standard checklists used for the person's specific cancer, whole person care reinforces and supports basic health behaviors, as described in Chapter 4, and using tools collected in Chapters 11 and 12.

PLANNING FOR SURVIVORSHIP

Of course, people living with a history of cancer need ongoing care. Guidelines from the NCCN suggest care should include[6]:

- Surveillance for cancer spread or recurrence; screening for subsequent primary cancers
- Monitoring long-term effects of cancer, including physical and psychosocial effects
- Prevention and detection of late effects of cancer and therapy
- Evaluation and management of cancer-related syndromes, with appropriate referrals for targeted intervention
- Coordination of care between primary care providers and specialists to ensure that all of the survivor's health needs are met

The Usual

Some clinics provide a survivorship care plan (SCP) according to older (pre-2020) Commission on Cancer directives, and some don't. We know this plan as a record of a patient's cancer treatment history, as well as a schedule of checkups and follow-up tests the person needs in the future. SCPs list possible long-term effects of the treatment or red flags for the person to watch for, along with suggestions for preventive measures.

In Jan's case, despite curative intent therapy for multiple cancers over many years before 2020, she never received a SCP. This is not uncommon. Without a well-integrated EHR, any such document is onerous for care teams to complete. It often only contains boilerplate language about standard health practices such as eating so many servings of vegetables a day, exercise, and cancer screenings that have been previously communicated to the person in other settings, such as primary care.

Data shows the questionable impact of the practice of SCPs. The process remains mostly a "push" of information to a patient-survivor, without space or request for input from the whole person. Typically, there isn't much or any motivational interviewing or health coaching in this realm of SCP creation.

The Possible

Survivorship visits, clinics, and care plans are informed by the actual person living with or beyond the cancer. This is where a HOPE visit can take center stage. Inviting a person in survivorship to complete a Personal Health Inventory (PHI), even if one had been completed earlier in the process, can allow what matters *now* to lead the discussion. A HOPE visit gives a way for the person to see their own path forward, vetted with a trusted professional. With good integrated EHR use, the conversation becomes visible to their primary care provider or other physician (for example, gynecologist, neurologist, cardiologist, etc.). A frank discussion about the myriad of internet claims about recurrence prevention can occur, using the Four Ps model as a guide (see Chapter 6 for more on the Four Ps).

The standard survivorship template is useful for giving the person with cancer a concise record to share with other providers, but it typically provides information without including any input from the person it's meant for. The person may not be asked about their preferences for survivorship care, for example. A survey of women who had been treated for early breast cancer showed that they wanted their primary care physician to help them with comorbidity treatment and general preventive care but wanted their oncologist to handle mammography screenings and ongoing cancer surveillance.[7] This lack of personalization and patient input to SCPs may be why a 2019 meta-analysis of such plans found they resulted in scant difference on patient's self-reported outcomes for factors like physical functioning and anxiety 12 months later.[8]

In whole person cancer care, survivorship visits, clinics, and care plans are informed by the actual person living beyond the cancer. Revisiting or initiating a PHI at this point can help the person form a larger perspective on their care going forward. If the PHI has been used earlier in cancer care, say during initial treatment, the ability to compare answers from then to now can highlight for the person their strength and the movement toward what is possible, based on their input, in their healing process now. Invitation of the person's perspective at this transition of care may ameliorate what is often described by survivors as a period of feeling lost without the care team. Ringing the bell (as is done in some clinics) at the end of treatment is a signal that one phase has ended but can also be the signal of the next step—survivorship and a return to wellbeing. This could be a moment to schedule a HOPE visit as something empowering for patients to look forward to during a possibly uncertain time.

BEYOND THE BELL (AND THE BOILERPLATE)

Whole person cancer care goes beyond the boilerplate language and standard health recommendations of a basic survivorship plan. Dietary and lifestyle changes and complementary therapies have been shown to help improve the health and wellbeing of cancer survivors, help prevent recurrence, and even extend lifespan.[9] The end of treatment is a transitional time when people may be more open to lifestyle changes, especially if they are convinced that the changes will help them avoid recurrence, improve function, and postpone death. Care teams can learn to apply a whole person approach to educate and help people overcome barriers. Engage every resource that makes sense, even if not taken up by the person during initial diagnosis and treatment. Teams offering support in survivorship do so by acknowledging a person's inherent ability to heal. You might even tell a person how their strength has been apparent throughout treatment, how you see they are healing now. Their strength can be put to making them even healthier than they were before cancer, a desire we often hear from patients who have been empowered by the challenge cancer presented them.

Food as Pharmacy

A number of good studies have shown that sticking to the ACS dietary recommendations for breast cancer (maintain a healthy weight, avoid alcohol, follow a healthy diet with at least 5 servings of fruits and vegetables a day, whole grains, lean protein, and low-fat dairy) is associated with reduced risk of recurrence and death among long-term survivors.[10,11] Many similar studies have shown dietary interventions are helpful for almost all adult cancer survivors.[12]

When food is optimized for healing and is combined with regular exercise, the benefits for cancer survivors are even better. A study of stage III colon cancer survivors over a 7-year period found that those who followed the ACS dietary and exercise guidelines most closely had improved disease-free survival and a 42% lower risk of death. The improvement in mortality risk from diet and exercise is larger than from most chemo-prevention studies, yet we usually prescribe drugs more than behavior change.[13] Why? A study that looked at adherence to the ACS cancer prevention lifestyle recommendations in women before, during, and 2 years after treatment for high-risk breast cancer found that people who had the highest adherence to the guidelines reduced their risk of recurrence by 37% compared to the people with the lowest adherence. Additionally, the highest-adherence group reduced their risk of death by 58%, compared to the lowest-adherence group.[14]

Movement Is Medicine

Despite all the evidence for exercise as a way to help with cancer-related health issues during and after treatment such as fatigue, quality of life, and physical function, and despite authoritative guidelines from the American College of Sports Medicine (ACSM),[15] research shows the majority of people living with and beyond cancer are not regularly physically active. It could be that this was true for the person prior to diagnosis, so suggesting movement as medicine may require significant health coaching for behavior change. In survivorship, care teams can refer people to home-based or community-based exercise or to outpatient rehabilitation, as appropriate.

This may require teams to truly believe the science that movement is medicine and to overcome some old beliefs. For example, for many years we were told that women with lymphedema shouldn't exercise. We now know that for women experiencing lymphedema or at risk of it, exercise is not only safe but also preventive.[16] To get there, we may need to educate ourselves on the benefits. In other words, our engagement, and not just patients' engagement, is needed when behavior change is required.[17]

Some cancer survivors find that returning to physical activity on their own is difficult. Here it helps to widen the team. For example, the care team can write an exercise prescription for working with a physical therapist, rehab specialist, or trainer at a rehab gym or community-based gym. We can make referrals to Livestrong at the YMCA, a free program led by trained instructors. The program adheres to ACSM guidelines for survivors engaging in exercise and consists of 2, 90-minute sessions a week for up to 12 weeks; it includes a complementary family membership for 12 weeks.[18]

Other wellness factors described in Chapter 4 and tools provided in Chapters 12 and 13 can assist in optimizing survivorship visits.

ADDRESSING LONG-TERM SIDE EFFECTS

Lingering side effects of treatment can seriously impact the activities of daily living and quality of life for survivors. Whole person care and integrative approaches can be utilized in concrete ways that make a difference for those ongoing problems.

Pain

Ongoing pain from surgery, chemotherapy-induced peripheral neuropathy, and other treatments (and aging) is very common in people with a history of cancer.[19] Nearly 35% of cancer survivors report having chronic pain, or pain on most days or every day in the past 6 months—a rate that is nearly double that for the general population. About 1 in 6 cancer survivors report having high-impact chronic pain, or pain severe enough to limit daily activities.[20]

People with pain aren't always getting the help they need. A study in 2019 found that 30 to 50% of patients with breast or colorectal cancer weren't talking to their doctors or getting advice about pain. The researchers found that only about 58% of people with pain were getting help for it.[21]

Using complementary modalities with or instead of pharmaceuticals to help pain can be effective and can lead to better sleep, better quality of life, less use of pain medication, and fewer health care appointments. The joint SIO–ASCO guideline for pain management is an excellent guide to evidence-based recommendations on integrative approaches to managing pain in patients with cancer.[22] The strongest recommendations are acupuncture and yoga for aromatase inhibitor–related joint pain; guided imagery, acupuncture, reflexology, or acupressure for general cancer pain or musculoskeletal pain; and massage for pain during palliative or hospice care.

Gentle exercise such as tai chi or yoga can help with pain relief. Mind-body therapies and relaxation techniques such as cognitive behavioral therapy and meditation can also be helpful.

The science underlying these modalities are described more fully in Chapter 4 and tools to implement them are provided in Chapter 12; also see the Pocket Guide to Cancer Pain and other pain information on the Healing Works Foundation website.

Fatigue

Cancer-related fatigue (CRF) is an almost universal side effect of any cancer treatment. The impact often continues long after the treatment is over. Persistent fatigue seriously impacts quality of life and the ability to return to work. Many people say it is the worst cancer symptom.

The NCCN Cancer-Related Fatigue Guidelines Panel defines CRF as "a distressing, persistent, subjective sense of physical, emotional, and/or cognitive tiredness or exhaustion related to cancer or cancer treatment that is not proportional to recent activity and interferes with usual functioning. Compared with the fatigue experienced by healthy individuals, CRF is more severe, more distressing, and less likely to be relieved by rest."[23]

Sometimes CRF is related to pain, poor quality sleep (see below), nutritional deficiencies, or comorbidities. When these have been ruled out, we look to address the fatigue itself. CFR gradually improves over time for many people—patience is needed. In the meantime, naps and commonsense steps to conserve energy can be recommended. Steps to improve sleep, as discussed elsewhere in this book, will also help.

Although it seems a paradox to people experiencing fatigue, gentle physical activity has been shown to be helpful by many studies.[24] Movement through yoga,[25] tai chi, and qigong[26] also helps.

Massage therapy also has good evidence for effectiveness.[27] The evidence for acupuncture and acupressure is mixed, but these modalities are known to help with relaxation and pain, so they may be helpful for underlying causes of fatigue.[28] In fact, any intervention that helps with relaxation will probably also help CRF.[29] If someone is too fatigued to even consider gentle exercise, it could be that offering these modalities, done to the body rather than by it, can create a bridge back to activity.

Mindfulness-based stress reduction techniques have been shown to be helpful for persistent fatigue in cancer survivors. Relaxation techniques are an effective, simple, and low-cost tool to help—see Chapter 13 for more details on how patients can learn them.[30] Having people explore self-care without movement, but with the power of their own mind and intention, can further strengthen their inherent capacity to heal.

Sleep Disturbances

Sleep disturbances are a big contributor to CRF. Almost 40% of survivors report ongoing sleep problems 5 years after treatment ended. Pain, discomfort, and worries over finances and cancer recurrence are underlying causes of insomnia.[31] The same sleep hygiene measures discussed in Chapter 12 and elsewhere in this book can help with long-term sleep disturbances. Be sure to ask about sleep and fatigue in all follow-up appointments. Create a go-to list of reputable drugless approaches to share and for referral as appropriate.

Lymphedema

Lymphedema is a common problem postsurgery, especially when lymph nodes in the groin or armpit have been removed, but it can also occur in survivors of head and neck cancer. Fortunately, a number of good approaches help with lymphedema, including compression garments, massage, and exercise.

Compression garments can help reduce swelling, especially for the lower limbs and if venous insufficiency is also present. These garments should be properly fitted and customized to the patient to prevent restriction of circulation.[32]

Manual lymphatic drainage (MLD), a type of specialized massage, can help with lymphedema if done early in the course of its development. In moderate to severe lymphedema, MLD may not provide additional benefit. The methods should be performed only by a professionally trained therapist to prevent inadvertent damage to the area.[33]

As mentioned earlier in this chapter, research has shown that contrary to popular belief, exercise is not only safe but also preventive for people with or at risk of lymphedema.[34]

Brain Fog

Brain fog, more formally known as cancer-related cognitive impairment and informally called chemo brain, is a very real, very distressing, but little-understood side effect of chemotherapy. It affects about 75% of people during treatment and persists after treatment in about 35% of people.[35] The most common symptoms include memory, learning, and attention problems, along with language problems, slowed processing speed, and an inability to multitask. People with this side effect often say they feel foggy or absent-minded. Persistent or severe brain fog in older people may be related to age-related cognitive decline. Sometimes after treatment effects are subtle but noticeable to those closest to the person.

Jan, who before treatment had been the penultimate family trip planner, found herself making simple mistakes, like making a hotel reservation that began a month too early or booking a flight from the wrong airport. These mistakes distressed her until family members said they still wanted her to do the planning but would spot check the details. Subtle imbalance and vision changes occurred, which were not apparent (or checked out) until she fell off a single step she had not noticed once after a dinner out. Even though balance and eyesight changes were apparently common after her type of therapy, no one had warned her.

Complementary approaches include exercise (physical and mental), improved sleep, cognitive behavioral therapy, stress reduction by any means that works for the person and creating a structured environment to help with forgetfulness. None have strong evidence for effectiveness.

Tackling brain fog takes a multipronged approach from the care team. It's important to the person that it be taken seriously and not minimized or dismissed. Different approaches and combinations of approaches will help different people. We may reassure people that brain fog often improves or resolves within 6 to 12 months. To quell the related anxiety during that time, engaging people in any lifestyle, body, or mind-body practice of their choosing could prove helpful. Reassurance with actionable options may work better for some people than waiting alone.

EMOTIONS IN SURVIVORSHIP

While leaving active treatment is a milestone on the cancer journey, the emotions as someone rings the proverbial bell can be very mixed. Feelings of relief and joy at being alive can exist side by side with apprehension about the future and feeling cut off from the support of the care team. While a range of almost simultaneous contradictory emotions is normal, the experience can also be confusing and upsetting. For those on long-term or never-ending cancer-directed therapy, emotions ebb and flow.

Anxiety and Fear of Recurrence

The unfortunate reality about survivorship is that you don't know if you are a survivor until enough time has passed to feel like one. The 5-year survival timeline is driven by research custom, not biology. Not surprisingly, many (but not all) people with a history of cancer dread and fear recurrence and are anxious about their future. We help by carefully explaining what the signs and symptoms of recurrence are. Knowing what to look for can help people distinguish between normal aches and pains and signs that the cancer is coming back. For some, however, the nonspecific nature of many cancer symptoms becomes an ongoing source of worry. Over time, recurrence fears recede, but for some people they stay very near the surface of day-to-day experience for the balance of life, even after many healthy years.

Mindfulness meditation is a great tool for helping people cope with anxiety about recurrence and fears for the future. It has the additional benefit of helping people better handle other normal life stresses and worries. Jenny Leyh, a breast cancer survivor and patient advocate for the Healing Works Foundation, explains how helpful she found it:

> After close to a year of fighting cancer I was declared "cancer free." Although I was thrilled to reach the proverbial finish line, I found myself struggling to deal with the trauma that I had just experienced. I was physically beat up and emotionally struggling, and I felt almost as lost as I had when I was first diagnosed.
>
> I immediately went on a low-dose antidepressant, but that wasn't enough. Medication is a good first step, but I also needed to talk to someone about the complex emotions that I was feeling. I began to see a therapist and continued with yoga, acupuncture, and cannabis to combat both my physical and emotional pain. But the most effective thing for me in dealing with—and preventing—anxiety was the practice of mindfulness meditation.

Mindfulness meditation not only helps, but it's also easy to learn for those who have interest. Hospital systems, cancer centers, community organizations, and others often teach short, free or low-cost classes. People can also self-teach through the many sources found online. Inexpensive or free apps that teach meditation for self-calming and sleep, such as Calm or Headspace, are a good choice for self-teaching and self-managing a meditation practice. More information about meditation and relaxation techniques is found in Chapters 12 and 13 and on the Healing Works Foundation website.

Depression

Depression and anxiety are so common that the ASCO guidelines recommend we screen for them, starting at the time of diagnosis and continuing through treatment and recovery.[36]

Some factors may increase the risk for depression. People who feel abandoned or isolated after treatment is over, who are very fearful of cancer recurrence, who are experiencing financial or marital stress, or who have lingering physical side effects and pain may be more vulnerable. Some people express "survivor's guilt," feelings of guilt for surviving cancer when others they've known have not.

We can and do reassure people that there's no timetable for emotional recovery from treatment and adjustment to life afterward—and that any feelings of anxiety, depression, and guilt are within the normal response of people we have cared for. We can also be ready to refer to various modalities and professional treatment based on a compassionate response to what someone may be going through. Not everyone is open to talk therapy, cognitive behavioral therapy, or antidepressant medication. We can also be ready to educate patients (and ourselves) on the extensive evidence for exercise, sleep, social support, and mindfulness meditation to address mood disorders. Care teams with mental health and social work service integration are wonderful resources and a goal to consider for providing whole person care, as discussed in Chapter 3.

Intimacy

Adjusting to the new normal of life after treatment includes adjusting to changes in sexual health and intimacy. Many people struggle with body image, menopausal symptoms, painful intercourse, low libido, erectile dysfunction, concerns about fertility, and other issues. None of them have quick or easy answers.

Care teams can help by letting people know they can ask openly about their sexual concerns. Some people may be reluctant to bring up such personal issues. Asking tactfully may help them open up. When issues are raised, we can refer people as needed to medical professionals, such as urologists, fertility specialists, OBGYNs, and others with the expertise to help. Counselors may be able to help with relationship concerns. Support groups and cancer buddies can also be extremely helpful for venting about sexual problems and getting practical advice for dealing with them.

REMEMBER THE CAREGIVERS

The role of caregivers—and the stress they face—continues after treatment ends. A person with cancer needs time, support, and patience to regain physical and emotional health. In survivorship, the time toxicity of treatment lessens, but especially in the first year or 2 after treatment ends, the person usually has frequent follow-up visits, lab work, scans, and other appointments. Caregivers continue to help with activities of daily living. Financial issues persist if the person can't go back to work. At the same time, help from their larger social support network may decline. Caregivers still need the time and space to pay attention to their own medical and psychosocial needs, many of which had been tabled during their loved one's active treatment.

We can help by involving caregivers in the posttreatment planning, supporting them at follow up appointments, encouraging them to take time for themselves, and referring them for help where we can.[37]

GIVING BACK: WHAT SURVIVORS SAY

Many people with a history of cancer are eager to share their hard-earned experience and help others. For those interested in giving back, becoming peer counselors, cancer buddies, or support group participants are some ways to do so. Have someone on your team keep a list of opportunities for survivor volunteers in your hospital system, cancer center, and the larger community, to provide when people express interest. When Dr McManamon and a health communications researcher partnered survivors with medical students learning to use the EHR to complete SCPs informed by the patient voice, this is what patients said after participating:

- Empathy and listening are so important. We still need care *after* treatment.

- Learn more about patients' fears, hopes, what to say/what not to say to help us cope with the disease and survivorship.

- The diagnosis or label of cancer is not the sum total of me, and survivorship is not just the absence of cancer in my body and mind.[38]

One of Jan's most rewarding activities after cancer was to teach medical students about the patient experience and needs. During the COVID-19 pandemic she was able to do this all over the country through virtual group sessions with other patients.

Going Beyond: An Example

When Sue Weldon was diagnosed with breast cancer in 2004, she wanted to add complementary therapies to her conventional treatment. She quickly discovered that she was on her own—she found a lack of easily accessible resources on topics like nutrition, acupuncture, massage, yoga, counseling, and other ways for breast cancer patients to enhance their wellness and care for their emotional, spiritual, and physical needs. In 2009, Weldon founded Unite for HER to Help Empower and Restore others diagnosed with breast cancer. The program began in the

Philadelphia area and has since expanded to provide nationwide services, support, and education to those affected by both breast and ovarian cancers.

The mission of Unite for HER (www.uniteforher.org) is to enrich the health and wellbeing of those diagnosed with breast and ovarian cancers by funding and delivering integrative therapies. The organization now prioritizes outreach to underrepresented areas to help close the disparities gap in cancer treatment and after.

Today Unite for HER offers extensive wellness programs that educate patients about integrative cancer care and provide them with access to supportive services, such as acupuncture and massage, and resources such as care boxes and home delivery of fruits and vegetables, at no personal cost. The Wellness Passport Program, for example, provides up to $2,000 worth of integrative therapies and services free, without any cost to the person. The goal is to help people access these services and empower them to create their own integrative care plans.

In 2022, when Unite for HER surveyed 119 participating people with metastatic breast cancer, they found that integrative therapies were able to reduce stress, reduce medication given for side effects, and improve the reported quality of life.[39]

Sue says, "With the science and data behind our programs, we feel we can really move the needle on cancer care and integrative treatment. We work directly with nurse navigators at cancer centers to get people into our programs soon after diagnosis. The navigators initiate the conversation right at that point of care and explain why the person might want to partner with us. Our nutrition services are by far our most popular programs because food insecurity is a real issue for people with cancer in underserved communities. We help people get their basic needs met—which means we're also meeting the needs of their families and freeing up their resources for other necessities. We continue to innovate because we can't keep up with the needs." This is an example of an extended team helping patients get whole person care.

A NEW NORMAL

As you and your team think about how to innovate survivorship care, consider how to include the people you serve. New thinking by the team at the Ann B. Barshinger Cancer Institute at Penn Medicine in Lancaster, Pennsylvania developed a process for moving beyond survivorship to include wellness. They created an expanded team and consulted others, but used and supported their existing structure. As Penn Medicine's Dr Randall Oyer notes, "Calling the end of treatment 'survivorship' limited how the team thought about what mattered most to patients and what they needed." At an Integrative Oncology Leadership Collaborative (IOLC) conference, Dr Oyer and his team learned about the importance of wellness. He says, "My team knew that we needed a change. And once we dove into wellness, it was an aha moment. People knew that wellness is what our patients and we are working toward."

Consider what matters. Find out and let that guide your innovations into whole person cancer care.

SUMMARY POINTS

- A growing number of people are surviving and living with cancer for years.

- After successful treatment the challenges of cancer are not over. Pain, fatigue, brain fog, sleep disturbance, and emotional and intimacy challenges continue for most patients.

- These challenges as well as risk mitigation and general health promotion can be improved with whole person care. Good evidence exists for using nutrition, exercise, social and psychological support, and several integrative approaches to help with these challenges.

- The current approach to cancer survivorship planning is not effective. A redesign of our approach is needed to enhance wellness and whole person care is needed.

- Whole person care starts with what matters to the person to shape next step recommendations for recovery and remaining healthy.

- Examples and resources for whole person care after cancer treatment exist and are growing.

CHAPTER TEN

END OF LIFE

When it comes to diagnosis, or to death, we do our best to answer the questions, "Why?" "When?" and "How?" In doing so, especially when it will help a person approach the final phase of life, we carry out some of the most important work of our careers. It is not for the faint of heart. A pediatric hematology-oncology physician shares with colleagues the reactions he receives when others learn what he does for a living. These range from incredulous, "How can you do that?" to the honorific, "My hat's off to you. Thank you for doing what I could never do."

We suspect everyone in cancer care, from nurses to advanced practice providers and physicians, has experienced similar reactions. On a human level, we recognize this particular part of the cancer care trajectory, about who we must become to help people face what we all will. How we as care teams do this—be it with grace, distance, or something unique to the person we serve—can make all the difference in how a person transitions and how family and loved ones move forward after the loss.

The *what* of death is universal. The *when* is often elusive. The *why* is not as simple as the word "cancer" written on the death certificate. As each of her sequential cancers was found, the possibility of Jan's death reemerged. She "got her affairs in order" multiple times. She set up trusts, reviewed her will, logged her passwords, organized healing rituals, cleaned out her closet, updated the family photo albums, planned a trip, and told her husband she wanted him to go on with his life and find another love when she was gone. Then another treatment would be found. After the fourth cancer, this end-of-life ritual became rapid, routine, and unremarkable—for her. For others who cared for her it was still difficult. Jan faced her possible death straight on, but some people with cancer don't ever want to think of or plan for death, even down to the last minute of their life. This range of responses requires mental and emotional flexibility from the oncology team to meet people where they are. In this chapter we discuss issues that arise at the end of life and how attending to the whole person provides a solid basis from which to face the inevitable.

A GOOD DEATH

An old Chinese blessing wishes you a "long and healthy life, great happiness, and a good death." The last part is often forgotten in the modern medicine mindset that death is somehow a failure in the onslaught to cure. If there is a possible blessing often hidden in death by cancer as compared to a sudden heart attack, it is that we have more time for connecting with loved ones and for release of fear. Whether the time we have to create such comfort stretches out for only a few days or over months, the hospice model is attuned to helping people do that. A more protracted time allows for events such as life review (formal or otherwise), closure conversations, gift giving, making amends, and fulfilling final wishes. That place, if possible, is of a person's own choosing and company. There may be great healing during this time.

A friend of Dr Jonas cared for a nearby farm over many years. The friend discovered he had cancer only after it had spread widely throughout his body. He had only a few weeks to live. As Dr Jonas recalls:

Although he distrusted doctors and drugs, my friend often asked me if there was anything for pain and illness that didn't involve either of those or cost a lot. I would occasionally make suggestions and bring over some natural remedy patches for his arthritis. We would stand around and we would talk about people, the weather, and politics. A few days before he died, hospice was called in and a space for dying was created at home. Taking drugs for his pain was no longer an issue for him.

I went over to visit him, and we exchanged our mutual affection and gratitude for each other and our relationship. He reflected on how he had tried to work hard all his life, to always be honest, and how much he appreciated knowing me and knowing the land around us. Looking me right in the eye, he asked if I thought he had been an honorable man. I said he was and bid him farewell. As I was leaving, there was a line out the door of family and friends, each coming to say goodbye and to thank him for all he meant to the community. His life connected to so many others.

HOSPICE AND PALLIATIVE CARE

Hospice, a care model where comfort is the primary goal and active tumor treatment ceases for people who won't likely live for more than another 6 months, is increasingly available. It is often a blessing for those who are enrolled in time. Disparities in access remain especially in states where Medicaid expansion did not occur, for undocumented immigrants, and for people in rural settings.[1] Despite this, in modern oncology care, much of the actual dying occurs in hospice care rather than in our hospitals and certainly only unexpectedly in our clinics. Although hospice care is widely documented as being started too late for many, actual people living with cancer may not be ready to enroll within that 6-month window, particularly when they see options yet to try in terms of therapies.[2] Aggressive treatment in cases where there is little or no data on the benefits of continuing is partly driven by the continued fear, and by the language we bring to the "war" on cancer. That language encourages and admires the hero mindset of "fighting to the end," and to "never give up" with more surgery, more chemotherapy, more radiation in an already frail and ravaged body.

In 2023, the median length of hospice enrollment in the US remains under 3 weeks.[3] Retrospectively, we know that aggressive tumor-directed treatment near end of life is not life-giving. In fact, earlier access to palliative and comfort care and the option for less aggressive treatment prolongs both comfort and length of life—a more balanced approach to treatment and healing.[4,5]

But it is only in the period after any person's death that we can be sure of the timeline in reaching that endpoint. It's an inexact science, this extrapolation of clinical trial data to our own patients, many of whom would not have been eligible for the very trials that led to the last-line treatments we offer. Especially toward the end of life, our calculus requires integrating many variables: the person's age, degree of frailty or fitness, comorbid conditions, psychological and social fatigue, a desire not to be a "burden" on others, and their wishes in the face of most often unpalatable choices.

SPIRITUALITY

At the end of life, as we anticipate the loss of being together, social, emotional, and spiritual concerns may come to the forefront for the person with cancer. Although we don't often do so, studies have shown that patients want us to ask about their spiritual beliefs and appreciate when we do.[6] If we take the step of asking, and discover spiritual distress, we can refer sooner to our chaplain and palliative medicine colleagues for support. Care teams can be trained to ask pertinent questions, using tools such as the Faith, Importance and Influence, Community and Address (FICA) Spiritual History Tool. FICA includes questions such as, "Do you consider yourself spiritual or religious?" before moving into more open-ended questions that allow a team to honor and understand the person's wishes as care planning evolves more fully.[7] Linking the HOPE Note Toolkit process to these spiritual assessments is a way to make these discussions more common in routine practice.[8]

For over 20 years, Dr Ann Berger and the Pain and Palliative Care Team at the NIH Clinical Center in Bethesda, Maryland have looked deeply at the factors involved in healing. These factors overlap with tools we have suggested for use earlier in cancer care [Personal Health Inventory (PHI), HOPE Note Toolkit] and show that healing for the whole person need not start at the end of life, as is so often the case. Dr Berger's team developed and validated the NIH-HEALS, a 35-item, measure of psycho-social-spiritual healing.[9] NIH-HEALS allows needs assessment within 3 factors: 1. Connection—belief in and connection to a higher power, religion, religious community, and family; 2. Reflection & Introspection—finding meaning, purpose, gratitude and joy in nature, activities including those that connect mind and body, interconnectedness, present moment orientation, and an increased sense of awareness about the fragility of life; and 3. Trust & Acceptance—accepting what is, feeling resolved, feeling at peace, and trusting that caregivers, friends, and family will respond to needs as they arise. If the patient has had a HOPE visit at some point in their care, they will have already expressed to the team "what matters" to them in life and "what gives them joy," which are questions built into the, albeit shorter, PHI tool. This makes it easier to revisit those questions and open the conversation during what may be a more sensitive time, when hope for psycho-social-spiritual healing becomes paramount.

When a person makes the decision to move toward comfort measures and away from active treatment, priorities quickly shift. We have all seen, on the inpatient side, the rapid de-escalation of orders in the chart when a person elects transition to comfort care. No more 4:00AM lab draws (or any lab draws); vital signs discontinued. This shift often feels like a collective deep breath, a sense of relief that no one must meet the impossible task of staving off death. Interestingly, this opening is where the kindness, to which the team has always aspired, tends to rapidly fill the void left in the wake of active contingency planning. Pain control becomes paramount if it is the predominant concern. Other urgent matters, such as getting missing family members to the bedside, become the call to action.

INTEGRATIVE MODALITIES FOR A GOOD DEATH

In end-of-life care, the choice of integrative modalities can be driven solely by what the person would find interesting, pleasurable, or useful. Extensive services drawn from supportive care, complementary and alternative care, and spiritual care are offered by the Pain and Palliative Care team at the NIH. The work of their team shows the close alignment of palliative care and complementary care modalities, both during active treatment and at the end of life.

Not everyone wants massage, but for some it can be of real benefit as they face the end. For those who do not want to be physically touched, bioenergy techniques such as Healing Touch or Reiki, frequently discounted during conventional treatment, are often part of hospice care and can be offered to inpatients even before a transition to hospice.[10] Even though the word "touch" is in the name, in these practices such as Therapeutic Touch, Healing Touch, and faith-based laying on of hands, patients aren't actually touched. These modalities are often welcome and appear to be effective in relieving pain and anxiety.[11] Music therapy is another nontouch modality. It can be a simple offering of music, provided by trained volunteers, or a more formal session with a trained music therapist. Many complementary approaches, such as aromatherapy, guided imagery, access to nature, and spiritual care services are brought into end-of-life care, as they can and do provide comfort and well-being. As one of the largest collections of therapeutic modalities Dr Jonas has ever seen (in one setting), the palliative care service in the Clinical Center of the National Institutes of Health provides a hope-filled example. With proper planning, hospitals can provide such services even before the end of life.

In oncology, much of integrative end-of-life care occurs outside our purview. To be aware of its existence, and to support its use for the comfort of our patients, is to honor the ongoing humanity of the life trajectory that occurs outside the clinic and hospital walls.

THE PIVOT

Before people with cancer enter hospice care, oncology teams, the patient, and the family are almost uniformly focused on preventing death and prolonging survival. For care teams, personal and professional growth in the face of death may come with the realization that there is no failure in death. Dr McManamon had an experience where growth didn't come easily, but it came, just as death does, in the end:

> The man was young but old by the Army's standards; he had joined the service for financial stability. In his early 30s, he had completed the 10 weeks of basic training with some difficulty. Afterwards, he continued losing weight with increasing body pain and dysphagia. The pain was not responsive to NSAIDs, "given out like candy," he said, by the medics. When he was sent to me, a newly minted oncologist, I found he had widely metastatic esophageal cancer. At the time, I didn't even know that it was possible to occur like this in someone so young. His bony pelvis was particularly riddled. His family situation was complex: his young wife had mental health issues, they had 2 toddlers, marital strife, transportation issues, and absent extended family. He missed chemo appointments, quickly declined, and yet refused hospice.
>
> I left countless detailed messages on his voicemail, hoping we were just miscommunicating. I hoped that more clarity, more direction, more requests for a clinic visit could make everything OK. His final care episode in our community hospital came after his wife called 911 and the EMTs found him paraplegic

and pulling himself around their apartment on his emaciated belly, grunt-style. He was brought in for emergent radiation of spinal cord compression. His was the worst end of life I'd ever seen, even after a busy 3-year fellowship in Washington, DC.

And then came the thank you card. For what? I couldn't even look at it. It stood at attention on the break room table in pastel pink, mocking me. Over lunch, a nurse nudged it toward me, saying, "This is from his mom." And I started to cry inside, asking, "Why did she send this?" Said the nurse matter-of-factly, "She wanted to thank us for taking care of her son." It took some time, but I decided to let the thanks in. And I've let it in ever since, as hard as it is. Even hard deaths can help us grow if we will let them in.

When we are with people close to death who are not yet in hospice, commonly because they refused an earlier referral, often there is an abrupt pivot to hospice so they can die at home, should that be their stated wish. Although a person may have shared a "do everything" mindset up to this point, what is hoped for now has shifted drastically. We honor these evolving wishes. Quality metrics don't capture the whole person aspect of any one person's changing wishes. They say more about people's will to live and maybe less about hope, or the fear of taking away hope, than is widely cited. The changes near the end are easy to see but hard to study—they don't end up in the evidence-based pile of facts that are supposed to guide us. Suggestions that cancer care teams don't know how to offer palliative care and/or hospice early enough in the care trajectory ignore a parallel reality: the strength of any individual's sovereignty and right of refusal, and the complex dynamic of the social and spiritual forces in every human's life—and, in some places, the dearth of palliative care services.

When we state the risk versus the benefits of available therapies, and offer treatments supported by data, however imperfect, we may meet people where they are. But first, we must know where that is and what matters most to them. Time is needed for both the patient and the care team to figure that out. The importance of knowing what matters most, however, can't be overstated if we are to provide whole person cancer care. When we know what matters to the person and their family, the transition from treatment to palliation to end-of-life discussion is easier. We may ever so gently point out that at this juncture, the risk of side effects from any possible or proposed treatment and its chance of stabilizing the tumor (so-called progression-free survival, more accurately termed progression-free interval)[12] won't provide a cure and may not be in line with their stated hopes for the future. Based on such counsel, some patients shift to end-of-life care, hospice when appropriate; some do not.

Care that flows from a person's wishes can be a source of guilt for teams involved in cases that don't satisfy end-of-life quality metrics, such as chemotherapy given within 14 days of death (the official rate of that goal is for this to occur in less than 10% of cases). Abstractions of quality numbers do not always reflect the best care for any one person.

PLANNING FOR THE PIVOT

It is important to note studies have shown that advanced care planning conversations do not decrease hope in cancer care.[13,14] However, advanced directives aren't happening in cancer care to the degree they are needed.[15] For patients lucky enough to have a long-standing relationship with a primary care provider, encouraging an appointment to discuss advanced directives may be the most pragmatic route. This bypasses issues that may preclude discussions with the cancer care team and draws on a trust built over years. For patients without a primary care provider, or when that isn't practical, we must initiate the conversation. The reason we don't at the start may be that we don't want to take away hope at the very time we are planning treatment. Using a tool such as the FICA Spiritual Assessment up front could help us ease into advanced directive conversations with a basis of understanding the whole person. Research has shown that positive religious coping (or the belief that God is going to help and support you through difficulties) is associated with higher frequency of ICU care at end of life and lower completion of advanced directives.[16] We may have been asked (and taught) to engage with people on advanced directives and care planning without understanding their spiritual background. Asking about people's beliefs and wishes can make a difference in care.

STAYING IN THE NOW

At the end of life, staying in the moment is particularly important. To provide whole person care at the end of life means we admit we are in the actual place and time of anticipating death with them and their loved ones. It is a reaffirmation of commitment to care based on the person's terms. It is truly a way to offer dignity in care.[17] It stops the "doing to" and starts the "being with." It helps the pivot from curing to healing, something that the team doing whole person care may have been integrating all along the cancer journey.

To be sure, many people are clear and unwavering about their wishes from the time of a cancer diagnosis, particularly in private discussions with those of us on the care team. These people readily share their views on life and death and as the sole authority on themselves. We tend to listen and, to be honest, feel a sense of relief when someone is sure about the way they want to go forward. Although some relay feeling pressure from family members to "fight," others are in full alignment with their family's support from the beginning as to whatever trajectory they wish their care to take. In effect, champions of whole person care can acknowledge the opinions of all involved while stating, "Here, at this place and time, only the person's wishes matters."

DEATH IN CHILDREN

While cancer in children and adolescents is rare, it is still the leading cause of death by disease past infancy among children in the US. In 2021, an estimated 15,590 children and adolescents ages 0 to 19 had cancer (1 in 285 children) and 1,780 died of the disease in the US. Worldwide, the number of children diagnosed annually is estimated at 300,000.[18] Death in children is particularly hard on families and communities. Importantly, in 2010 the Patient Protection and Affordable Care Act required state Medicaid programs to pay for both curative, life prolonging treatment and hospice services for children less than 21-years old who qualify.

The management of the end of life for pediatric patients is beyond the scope of this book. However, as a family physician, Dr Jonas has dealt with his share of children's deaths. It can be challenging to get at what matters to the person when, at times, they are too young or sick to engage without a proxy. The family, parents, and siblings are lifelines to what matters for the dying child. What constitutes a "good death" occurs in the cocoon of a family's anticipatory grief. Teams in this situation give particular attention to issues of bereavement that follow. In the situation of children, the hope for a long life is gone, but the goals of peace and comfort can still occur during the life remaining.

For readers interested in the special needs of children and their families at the end of life, we refer you to the excellent guidelines provided by the American Academy of Pediatrics.[19]

AFTER DEATH: THE LIVING

People say that oncology care teams do things they could never do because we open ourselves to a world that regularly includes grief and loss. Or not. Sometimes we shield ourselves from those exposures, or we find ways to cope that may or may not bring joy in practice. With maturity and time, most of us on cancer care teams reach our own conclusions on how best to handle the death of people we care about, day in and day out.

Much remains unprocessed. Our training does not suggest ways of being productive in work while also making room for the grief and loss inherent in cancer care. Compartmentalizing is typical because it partly works. We get things done. The chart notes get written. But what best honors our wholeness as people who care? Consider ways your team may find meaning in work through honoring what we are actually doing as people who provide care. Doing so allows the people on your team to not only function at a time of loss, but to do so as whole people. Considering new ways of being with people and families facing end of life requires a commitment to remaining open, present, and whole. By naming and sharing these struggles we acknowledge the vulnerability and helplessness we all feel when someone we cared for dies.

There are many ways to assist the patient, family, oncology teams, and clinicians during this transition. Ignoring it is one way, but probably not the best in most circumstances. It leaves us "unwhole." Examples of ways to fill this hole include small but meaningful steps. When a person transitions to hospice care, for example, a team member makes direct contact with them or a designated family member, as appropriate, to wish them all well and to relay any personal best wishes—every time. Family members often want to inform people who were important in their loved one's care about their death. Opening a pathway to that act helps with closure on all sides and can be activated when they call in, as they often do, to cancel future appointments, or to let us know of the death.

BEING THERE

It has been said that people fear abandonment more than death. We can mitigate that fear by having someone from the team be in contact, or even better, be at the death if the patient and family request it. A close patient advocate can be the bridge to this event. The patient's primary care team may also be a bridge. Another step the care team can take upon learning of a person's death is for a clinic's designated representative to send a sympathy card to the family. What about this as a metric? Could your team follow something that matters to people at end-of-life care on a systematic basis? The card can be signed by as many care team members as wish to, as a way to acknowledge the relationship that was present up to death and the importance of the person now gone.

In team meetings or huddles, care team leaders can take a moment to state out loud the names of patients lost in the past month, as a touchstone to our work's meaning and the impact of the end of relationships on care team members themselves. This is a good time to remind team members of the designated point of contact within the institution (or on site) for cancer care team support in bereavement, as and when needed. No one should be abandoned in the process of end-of-life care, not even us.

As a first step, consider talking in your teams about why any of the above bereavement practices are not happening, what might be a better fit where you work, and whether they would help connect you all together to the thread of life we're trying to honor by the work we do in cancer care.

Clinicians and providers cite a lack of training in providing bereavement support as a real barrier to the very human function of reaching out to grieving loved ones following a patient's death. Teams need training—or to learn from the nonphysician members of our teams. In a 2020 study of US head and neck cancer surgeons (156 respondents; 18% response rate), nearly 70% cited being unaware of a patient's death; 50% cited a lack of mentorship/training in this area as barriers to bereavement practices such as making a phone call to the family or sending a letter.[20]

In 2010, a similar-sized cohort of cancer care providers in the Pacific Northwest (medical and radiation oncologists, surgeons, and palliative care or hospice physicians), responded to a survey on the most common perceived barriers to bereavement follow up. They cited lack of time and uncertainty of which family member to contact. Sixty-nine percent didn't feel that they had received adequate training on bereavement follow up during postgraduate training.[21] If your institution has a formal bereavement program, you are ahead of the curve. If you are looking to develop one, Dana-Farber Cancer Institute published on their experience in 2015 and provide guidance on doing so.[22]

SIGNS

In addition to the basic self-care items that we recommend for family and caregivers—get some sleep, make sure to eat, get away for a while—the survivors often continue to look for meaning. Meaningful signs from the unconscious or unknown side of spirituality often emerge around and after the end of life. Those who care for the dying say that these events happen routinely, because the human need to make meaning and transcend the self during and after death goes on. Between 30 to 50% of US adults (when given permission to safely talk) will tell about how a loved one visited them or showed them a sign after death, often to comfort and reassure them that they were all right. As military physicians, we often heard such stories from veterans who lost buddies in battle. Studies have shown that such experiences are common.[23] These visitations can be extremely healing if they are listened to with compassion and not overt skepticism or dismissal.

After Dr Jonas's father died, his wife of 60 years had a clear and startling visitation from him. She described in detail how she saw him, spoke to him, and held his warm hand. He told her he was always with her and would make sure she was taken care of for the rest of her life. Soon after that event, her grief and depression began to lighten, allowing her to go on with life. For the materialists reading this book, a growing body of evidence suggests that these near-death and after-death events are not just hallucinations or delusions.[24] For the curious, we recommend reading up on this extensive literature.

Other and more subtle signs of meaning occur when looked for. Dr Jonas recalls a cancer patient who was on life support with no chance of recovery:

> Because I had been her primary care physician, the family asked the oncology team to contact me, requesting that I be present when they turned off her life support, which I gladly did. I stood with them during her last breaths. On my way back from the hospital, I stopped in a park and walked

to the edge of a favorite stream. While sitting nearby, listening to the water and my mind largely blank, a beaver climbed up on a rock right in front of me. Totally unconcerned, it looked at me for a few minutes and then continued on its way. Weeks later, I received a stuffed toy beaver in the mail from her family, with a thank you note. It said that her favorite animal was the beaver, so they decided to send out some toy beavers to a few friends and caregivers. I had not known this about her nor discussed my experience at the stream with them. Those who work closely with the dying frequently tell stories about signs like this.[25]

HEALING THE HEALERS

Isolation of the sick and dying during the COVID-19 pandemic brought into stark focus the tragic suffering produced when loved ones cannot actually be there at the time of death. Many health care workers had to be stand-ins or hold the phone as people said their last goodbyes.

These deaths do not just pass *over* the care team, no matter how resilient they are. These deaths pass *through* them. After, accepting assistance from chaplains or counselors is team leadership.

Hospital chaplains often serve a role in helping to heal the healers. When Dr Jonas's daughter was serving as a hospital chaplain at Yale New Haven Hospital, she would keep an eye out for and offer support to the care teams and staff. After one particularly prolonged and failed attempt by multiple clinicians and team members to keep a young child alive, she offered those who had been involved in the child's care the opportunity to gather and do a short ritual, acknowledging the effort and expressing their feelings of letdown and grief. The experience was cathartic and brought the participants closer together, accelerating their recovery after such a collective trauma. One ICU nurse said the ritual not only helped her deal with that child's death but made her realize she had lots of pent-up grief from many deaths that, in her mind, were represented by the experience. For months after the ritual, care team members were able to talk more openly about the stresses and traumas their job immersed them in regularly. Why not have chaplains offer these rituals on a regular basis?

Opening opportunities for periodic rituals and discussions that allow teams to process the ongoing stresses and emotions that arise from the loss and traumas of cancer care could be a routine part of oncology, with chaplains and other support staff leading. While most oncology teams call a chaplain at the request of a patient or family member, surveys show that hospital chaplains often spend 30% or more of their time attending to staff support.[26] Given the rise in burnout and the frequency of death in oncology, maybe it should be even more.

DEATH AS CLOSURE

A death approaching is no less complex than the life that follows. Dr McManamon recalls a remarkable experience of closure:

> Years after a woman received adjuvant chemo-therapy from one of my colleagues, she was back, now a mother and facing metastatic cancer. She fought hard to remain on chemotherapy but had many of the complications that limit later lines of therapy. Still, she wanted treatment any way she could get it so she could live to see her firstborn's wedding; we pushed the envelope on blood count parameters, proceeding more aggressively, for a time. The cancer progressed, and she refused hospice despite transitioning off chemotherapy. Her partner, a trained medic, provided expert care and brought her in for periodic clinic visits. They looked more depleted by the week. After many months of having worked as a solo oncol-ogist, I welcomed a new partner and soon after headed to a much-needed family vacation. On day

3, standing in a noisy playground in Orlando, I received a call from my new colleague. My patient was in the hospital and not doing well; they were moving to comfort care.

Two days later, following my morning clinic, I made my way to her bedside and for the first time met her brother and elderly parents. Her spouse, the consummate caregiver, quickly ushered me to his seat at her head. She was alive but unresponsive. I held her closest hand as he took the one opposite. We spoke of her life and then she died hands in ours. After her family members hugged her torso and cried over her face and kissed her scalp, there were no more words. Only then did I fall back to the rites of listening to her chest and looking into her eyes, then closing them, carrying out the ritual not done since my internal medicine residency many years before. As an oncologist, I find myself so far removed from death that this happening seemed novel and ancient. And I see that she was in charge all along, and that I honored her wishes more than not.

Months later, her medic spouse came to see me. He wanted to give me something, and proceeded to press a heavy, embossed challenge coin into my hand, emblazoned with his prior office symbol and rank—a token of great value in military culture. I read aloud from the words held in my hand, about the promise of care by medics in his unit. I was deeply moved. He told me that a few months before she died, he lost his favorite pair of sunglasses. They looked everywhere, turning the house upside down, but couldn't find them. For his birthday, she gave him a new pair, but they weren't the same (the old ones weren't being made anymore). A few days prior, he got into his truck and saw, sitting right below the speedometer, his lost pair of sunglasses. Standing with me in the exam room, he began to weep. We held together while he sobbed. As we separated, he concluded she was telling him she's OK and that he can finally stop worrying about her.

Closure comes in many forms. Now, above my desk at home, this coin occupies 1 of 4 carved slots in my military US folded-flag display case, a reminder that we are all OK, always, somehow.

SUMMARY POINTS

- Helping patients and their loved ones have a "good death" is as complex as trying to keep them alive.

- Care teams are not well trained in dealing with the end. Preparing for the end early helps everyone when the time comes.

- Hospice and palliative care offer benefits at the end of life but are not used often or early enough.

- Supportive care, integrative care, and spiritual care have great utility at the end of life.

- Social support and the opportunity to make meaning of life are important for both the dying and the living.

- Death does not pass over the care team, it passes through them, so time, ritual, and space are needed for them to process death also.

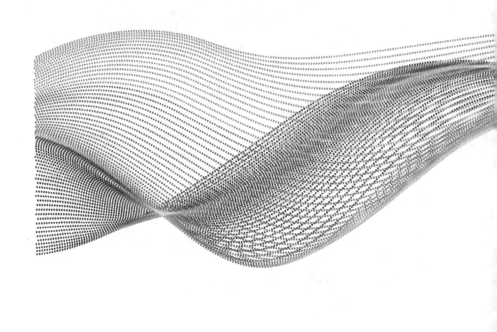
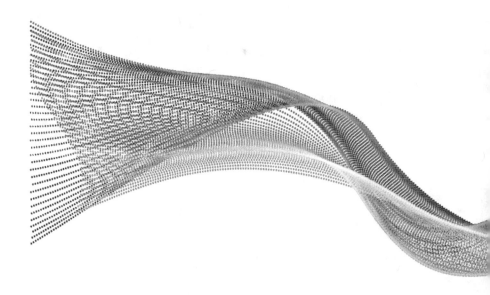

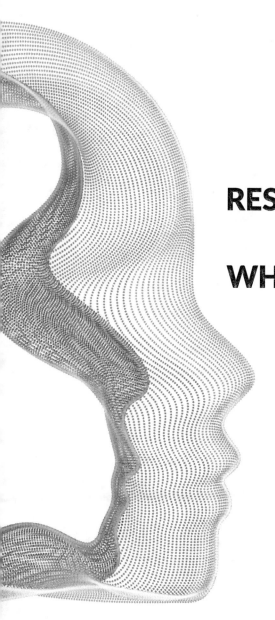

PART THREE

TOOLS AND RESOURCES FOR DELIVERING WHOLE PERSON CARE

CHAPTER ELEVEN

DOING A WHOLE PERSON CARE VISIT

Doing whole person care requires setting aside time for the team to talk and plan with the person with cancer about what matters to them and incorporate wellness, integrative, supportive care, psychological support, and social needs into the plan. The ideal approach is to schedule a visit in which these factors are the main focus. However, some teams add this discussion into part of a standard or extended cancer treatment visit. Either way, the team and the patient need to take the time and have the tools to explicitly have these discussions.

In addition, the patient needs a good understanding of what whole person care means, how it's done, and what their role is during the cancer treatment and healing journey. Because many elements of whole person care aren't routinely part of what oncology teams provide (or patients expect), discussing it with the patient and discerning their needs is a process involving several steps. We start by introducing the topic to the patient and providing them with information about it. They are asked to provide information about their needs and desires. Time at a specific visit (or set aside in or around a regular visit) is dedicated to discuss these and to describe the resources available to them as the cancer is treated. After the initial plan is mutually agreed upon, revisit it periodically (things change) to keep what matters at the center of discussion and modify the plan as needed.

Organizing and training the care team can greatly facilitate these discussions and reduce the time needed for whole person care. So can having the right tools at your fingertips. In the Integrative Oncology Leadership Collaborative (IOLC), 12 centers met on a monthly basis over 2 years to develop, discuss and test a set of tools designed to make whole person care more routine. Those tools were collected into a Healing-Oriented Practices and Environments (HOPE) Note Toolkit and are on the Healing Works Foundation website. IOLC sites used these and other tools they had to advance whole person care. While there are many ways to do whole person care, we thought that showing the details of how one clinic uses the HOPE Note Toolkit would be useful for readers. This chapter explains those tools and resources, gives ideas for implementing them, and illustrates how they are being operationalized in a practice. We will start with a story about a patient leader in the IOLC and how she integrated these approaches into her own care.

JENNY

Jenny Leyh shared in Chapter 9 how she tapped into healing after cancer. But let's rewind to May 2016 when she was 33 and in the third trimester of pregnancy when diagnosed with triple negative breast cancer, stage IIB. "After the initial shock wore off, I was determined to fight the cancer with everything I had," says Jenny. Along with her conventional cancer treatments, Leyh used multiple modalities to stay strong during and after treatment, to relieve her anxiety and to minimize treatment side effects.

Doctors at Johns Hopkins Medicine recommended chemotherapy before surgery to help combat the cancer without harming her baby. The molecules in the chemotherapy are too large to cross the placenta, her doctors explained. Her medical oncologist worked closely with her OBGYN to develop her cancer treatment plan and monitor Jenny's baby until she was safely born in June 2016.

Over the next year and more, Jenny completed 16 rounds of chemotherapy, followed by a bilateral mastectomy with tissue expanders and breast implants and radiation therapy. But as each round of chemotherapy shrank her tumor, the harsh treatment also wrought havoc on her body. She had joint pain, debilitating fatigue, tender fingernails and toenails, and a general flu-like feeling.

When Jenny had difficulty lifting her daughter due to back pain and stiff joints, she knew she had to take action. Instead of the pain medications her doctor prescribed, which caused more side effects, she turned to gentle yoga and acupuncture. Getting light exercise regularly and eating a healthy, mostly plant-based diet improved her overall wellbeing.

Her doctors told Jenny she was cancer free in April 2017. But like many cancer survivors, she still had late effects from her treatments and was worried about her cancer coming back. "The combination of low-impact exercise, meditation, therapy, cannabis, and the antidepressant helped me through some dark times," she says.

Jenny had to pull her whole person care together on her own, as so many patients do. She was intelligent, had resources, and had a fierce and active advocate in her husband. Together they created a plan and adapted it as they went along. Today, Jenny has 2 lovely children and works as a journalist and patient empowerment specialist. She knows that many patients can do what she did—and more—preferably with some assistance from their oncology teams.

As leader of the IOLC Patient Advocacy and Empowerment Collaborative (PAEC), she has written and built many of the resources discussed in this part of the book and has had major input into making these tools patient friendly. Jenny led the PAEC group to review the HOPE Note Toolkit items and provide feedback. She and other PAEC members reviewed the resources such as the

Pocket Guides (short topical summaries), patient guides, videos, and intake tools (for example, Personal Health Inventory [PHI]) from a patient perspective. These resources are now available free for use in any practice and can be found and downloaded from the book website (www.HealingandCancerBook.com) or readers can go to a special landing page that features the resources and tools for patients (https://howwehealcampaign.com/resources/cancer/).

WHEN TO DO A WHOLE PERSON CARE VISIT

Not all patients are as educated, engaged, and empowered as Jenny, especially after they first get a diagnosis of cancer. Multiple discussions during IOLC sessions explored the best time to delve into whole person care with patients. All agreed that whole person care was needed throughout the cancer journey and that there were specific times where those discussions were most appropriate. Jenny believes a separate visit to address the issues in whole person care is the ideal way to approach patients. Many systems inserted whole person care topics into routine sessions.

Most IOLC members agreed that the first visit following diagnosis is not usually the time to begin these discussions. At that point, patients are often anxious, confused, and looking for a definitive cancer treatment plan. Once the treatment plan is in place and the person with cancer has the capacity to think more about other matters, discussions about wellness, self-care, and supportive and integrative approaches become feasible. Finally, all IOLC members agreed that whole person care discussions are needed after treatment and in survivorship planning, empowering patients in methods to improve wellbeing and prevent relapse. Regardless of when these discussions happen, following a defined sequence of steps—the previsit, the visit, and the follow up—increases the likelihood that whole person care will occur. For teams that would like to use the HOPE tools, designed to support each step in the sequence, we describe them and how we use them on the following page.

THE HOPE NOTE TOOLKIT

Care teams can use the HOPE Note Toolkit to prepare and plan for each phase in the sequence. The HOPE Note Toolkit contains the following:

- PHI
- A Whole Person Health visit guide and the HOPE Note
- Personalized Health Plan (PHP)
- Related resources individualized for the person with cancer

The HOPE Note Toolkit was originally designed for use in primary care and was tested in 16 primary care centers around the US.[1] The 12 cancer centers in the IOLC then created, tested, and refined versions of the tools for use in cancer care. Examples of how these and other centers are doing whole person care are summarized in Chapter 15. The HOPE tools are described below.

The Personal Health Inventory

The PHI is a patient-facing questionnaire used by oncology care teams to quickly show a patient what whole person cancer care is. It's used to elicit feedback on what matters to the patient as a person, and what they need to feel whole. Adapted from a questionnaire for use in the VA, it shows the oncology team what to focus on to help support the patient's health and wellbeing. Patients usually fill out the PHI before a whole person care visit, sometimes called an integrative health visit or for part of the discussion during a regular visit.

The PHI starts by explaining whole person care, asking about current health status using Likert scales for physical, mental, and overall wellbeing. Teams may also want to use a validated assessment of a patients' current health status through questionnaires like the FACT-G7 (Functional Assessment of Cancer Therapy—General—7 Item Version) or the ESAS (Edmonton Symptom Assessment Scale).[2] Note: the FACT-G7 does require licensure (at no cost for clinical use but permission required)—please see requirements (https://www.facit.org/measures/FACT-G7).

This personal health inventory is adapted from
and aligned with the VA's Whole Health model.   PATIENT'S NAME: _____   DATE: _____

Personal Health Inventory

Complete your personal health inventory before your integrative oncology visit. We'll use this to discuss how you can enhance your health and well-being during and after treatment of the cancer.

Use this circle to help you think about your whole health.

All areas are important and connected to your ability to heal and be healthy.

- The outer ring addresses what your home and work are like and how you feel physically.
- The next ring addresses everyday choices on self-care and lifestyle.
- The social and emotional ring looks at your relationships and social support.
- The inner ring addresses **what matters** to you most and brings you joy and meaning in life.

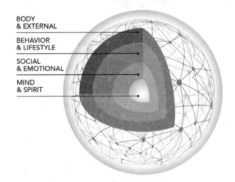

BODY
& EXTERNAL

BEHAVIOR
& LIFESTYLE

SOCIAL
& EMOTIONAL

MIND
& SPIRIT

Rate where you feel you are on the scales below from 1-5, with 1 being poor and 5 being excellent.

	Poor	Fair	Good	Very Good	Excellent
Physical wellbeing	◯ 1	◯ 2	◯ 3	◯ 4	◯ 5
Mental/emotional wellbeing	◯ 1	◯ 2	◯ 3	◯ 4	◯ 5
Life: How is it to live your day-to-day life?	◯ 1	◯ 2	◯ 3	◯ 4	◯ 5

Figure 11.1 Oncology-specific Personal Health Inventory – Page 1

Cancer-sensitive language was adjusted from the version of the PHI used in primary care by the IOLC. See text for and explanation of its parts and use.

What do you live for? What is most important for you in your life? What brings you joy?

Write a few words to capture your thoughts:

What do I need to know about you as a person to give you the best care possible?

Where You are Now

Write in a number between 1 (poor) and 5 (excellent) that best represents where you are now. Then please mark up to three items you would like to work on.

Area of Whole Health	Where I am now (1–5)	Pick up to three items
BODY & EXTERNAL		
Feeling safe: Having comfortable, healthy spaces where you work and live. The quality of the lighting, color, air, and water. Decreasing unpleasant clutter, noises, and smells.		
Paying for Basics: Quality and availability of food, housing, utilities, and transportation.		
BEHAVIOR & LIFESTYLE		
Moving: Moving and doing physical activities like walking, dancing, gardening, sports, lifting weights, yoga, cycling, swimming, and working out in a gym.		
Sleep: Getting enough rest, relaxation, and sleep.		
Food: Eating healthy, balanced meals with plenty of fruits and vegetables each day. Drinking enough water and limiting sodas, sweetened drinks, and alcohol.		
SOCIAL & EMOTIONAL		
Social Support: Feeling listened to and connected to people you love and care about. The quality of your relationships with family, friends and people you work with.		
Stress Management: Tapping into the power of your mind to heal and cope. Using mind-body techniques like relaxation, breathing, or guided imagery.		
MIND & SPIRIT		
Purpose: Having a sense of purpose and meaning in your life. Feeling connected to something larger than yourself. Finding strength in difficult times.		
Learning and Growing: Developing abilities and talents. Balancing responsibilities where you live, volunteer, and work.		

PHI-Cancer-V2

Figure 11.2 Oncology-specific Personal Health Inventory – Page 2

The PHI asks what patients most enjoy and live for (what matters), and then asks them to rate where they are on a 1 to 5 scale in the following areas:

- Physical environment
  - Feeling safe
  - Paying for basics
- Lifestyle and behavior
  - Moving
  - Food
  - Sleep
- Social and emotional
  - Stress
  - Social support
- Mental and spiritual
  - Life purpose
  - Learning and growing

Through the graphic on the PHI, the team can quickly communicate to the patient the main components of whole person care. The PHI provides a way to get a snapshot of where the person is in terms of health and wellbeing and what areas of support are needed. It usually takes patients 5 to 10 minutes to fill out. As mentioned in Chapter 6, the PHI and HOPE questions can be built into the EHR for patient convenience. It is also available to be fielded electronically through a low-cost, online HIPAA compliant survey platform, then uploaded in the EHR as a PDF. Or it can be completed on paper before any visit to rapidly pinpoint 1 or 2 areas outside tumor treatment that are important to the patient. We give examples of uses of the PHI later in this chapter.

The Whole Person Care Visit and the HOPE Note Toolkit

Using the PHI, the team then conducts a whole person care visit (some call it an integrative health or HOPE visit) and incorporates key questions from the PHI into the visit and documents the discussion. The documentation can be integrated with the standard Subjective, Objective, Assessment, and Plan (SOAP) note or as a stand-alone HOPE Note. In either case, the purpose is to envelop the cancer care within what the patient cares about and needs for better health and wellbeing.

HOPE NOTE QUESTIONS

What Matters:
- What is most important to you in life?
- What are the primary activities you want to retain during treatment?

Body and External:
- What is your home like?
- Your work environment?
- How often do you get out in nature?

Behavior and Lifestyle:
- How is your diet?
- How is your sleep?
- How do you manage stress?
- How is your activity level?

Social and Emotional:
- How is your social support?
- How was your childhood?

Spiritual and Mental:
- What are you most worried about?
- What brings you joy?
- What provides you with meaning and purpose?

Oncology care teams use the PHI and the HOPE Note during a whole person health visit to identify and address what matters most to the patient. This process helps engage the patient in shared decision-making about their health and healing, putting them front and center in the care plan. Teams offer evidence and support to help patients meet those goals.

The Personalized Healing Plan

During the first whole person health visit, the provider and patient work together to create a PHP, which is integrated into their cancer care. The PHP lists up to three things the patient wants to work on to live healthier and participate in what matters most to them. It also includes steps, resources, and team support for making progress in addressing their needs. Some patients say they want to do "everything" to treat their cancer, but that doesn't lend itself to effective change. Having them focus on their top 3 (or even top 1) will make it more likely they will be successful.

Resources and Support

Related resources created for whole person cancer care include the Integrative Oncology Solution Guide for providers and Pocket Guides for patients and providers (https://healingworksfoundation.org/whole-person-cancer-care). Multiple other resources are available and collected for use on the book website. Clinics can add and customize their own resources. A landing page with patient-ready materials that you can download and use to provide to patients can be found at https://howwehealcampaign.com/resources/cancer/. All these materials have been vetted by oncologists and patients in the IOLC and PAEC and with other subject matter experts.

The Integrative Oncology Solution Guide

The Integrative Oncology Solution Guide is a resource mapping tool developed with the IOLC to help providers conduct whole person health visits and address areas patients are ready to work on to improve and maintain their health. It can be found on the

Healing Works Foundation website. Providers can customize the guide for their cancer center by inserting active links to resources they most recommend and put them into usable formats for their workflow. The care team can use the guide to begin discussions with the patient and then click on the resource they want, such as educational handouts, technology links, referrals, or community resource links.

The guides cover 5 areas: nutrition, sleep, stress management, activity, and social support. The page on each area starts with the relevant HOPE Note questions and then lists recommended actions for care team to choose from in four categories:

- Educational handouts for self-care
- Technology
- Internal resource or specialist
- Community resources

Pocket Guides

Pocket Guides for patients and providers provide easy-to-read information about topics that are important to people with cancer. Most guides include information about behavioral and lifestyle treatments people can use to feel better. Some offer ways to cope with the physical and emotional side effects of cancer treatment. Evidence summaries of behavioral, complementary and integrative health care approaches, such as nutrition, activity, acupuncture and yoga, are provided. Each summary includes a description on how each approach is accessed and used, current training, licensing, payment information, and scientific evidence for their use.

Pocket guides are free for patients to download or teams to use and share with attribution. The currently available guides include these titles:

- Young Adult and Teen Cancer
- Financial Impact of Cancer
- Cancer and Sexual Health

- Cancer and Spirituality
- Nutrition and Cancer
- Movement and Cancer
- Cancer Pain
- Peripheral Neuropathy
- Supplements and Cancer
- Cannabis and Cancer

Others are being produced regularly. Contact us if you are interested in a Pocket Guide for an area you do not see on the website but use often. You can read and download the pocket guides (https://healingworksfoundation.org/whole-person-cancer-care/pocket-guides/).

THE WHOLE PERSON CARE PROCESS

How are the HOPE Note Toolkit and these resources used in day-to-day care? Here we describe a clinical care path for incorporating these tools into patient management. The visit process and care flow by the care team is illustrated in Figure 11.3 and briefly described below.

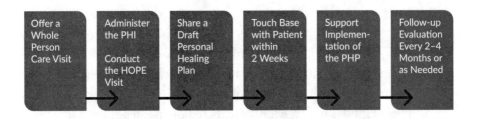

Figure 11.3 A Clinical Care Path for Whole Person Cancer Care

Delineated here is one way to integrate whole person care into an oncology practice. Chapter 11 describes how one clinic uses this care pathway to routinely deliver whole person care.

Screening

In this clinic, a nurse, advance practice provider, or navigator screens patient for their, needs, interest, and desire to engage in whole person cancer care by describing what it is, listing the related services available at the hospital/clinic, and asking if they have interest in learning more. If they do, the clinical team hands or sends them an information flyer on whole person care and asks them to read it or watch a video (https://vimeo.com/725685604).

If the person with cancer is ready to access and use these services, they make an appointment for a whole person cancer care visit through the regular appointment channels. If they're not interested, that information is noted. They may be asked again periodically, depending on their situation and progress or regress. Screening for interest is not required but allows choice for patients and appropriate use of resources.

Previsit Information

Once an appointment is made, the patient is sent the link to information on whole person care and a link to fill out the PHI. If they arrive for the visit and haven't completed the PHI, we request that they finish it in the waiting room prior to the visit.

The Visit

During the whole person care visit (or during the whole person discussion part of a regular visit), the team uses the PHI as a guide for the discussion. The clinician or team member uses open-ended questions about the primary issues the patient would like to address—in other words, the answers they gave on the PHI. Ideally, the visit should include a discussion of what matters. What is the patient's reason for wanting to engage in whole person care? The response is written at the top of the second page of the PHI. For example, if the patient says that family is the most important thing in their life, they are asked to talk more about their family and how treatment connects with or impedes goals they have related to family. How can their cancer care be adjusted to help them keep family goals attainable?

A look at the scores (1 to 5) at the bottom of the second page of the PHI indicates which areas to focus on during the visit. The lowest score becomes the highest priority for discussion and support services. A summary of the visit is recorded in the EHR using a routine documentation note or a HOPE Note template.

For example, if "sleep" is marked with a low score, the team asks more detailed questions about their sleep, such as problems with pain, daytime sleepiness, alertness, or frequent awakenings. They provide resources to assist with that area. If "basic needs" are inadequate, more detailed information is gathered on finances and social determinants of health and referrals appropriate to the situation are offered.

The Personal Healing Plan

At the end of the visit, a PHP is created that summarizes the action items from the visit. In Dr Jonas's clinic this includes the following items, adjusted as appropriate:

1. A treatment plan or list of options for the patient's main goal and/or area of greatest need (pain, for example) with specific recommendations. In the case of pain, the plan could include actionable steps, such as trying medications or supplements, acupuncture, breathing or mindfulness exercises or referral to therapeutic touch or medical massage.

2. A summary of any labs, referrals, informational and educational links, technology assists, or other recommendations designed to facilitate behavioral change.

3. A template form is filled out during the visit by the clinician, with items for the medical assistant to provide the patient at checkout that relate to areas of the initial PHP.

4. At checkout the medical assistant provides the patient with a checklist of next steps and information (such as a Pocket Guide) on the primary wellness, supportive, and integrative activities discussed. Follow-up appointments are made before they leave the clinic.

5. This is followed by a message with links to the same information and a thank-you note for the visit via the patient portal. Most of this can be automated.

6. An appointment for a follow-up phone call in 2 weeks is made with the trained medical assistant, nurse, APP, social worker, or health coach, to check in as to any questions from the resources provided (see below). In person follow up with the primary clinician or oncology team lead is in 1 to 3 months, or as appropriate.

Follow ups

In 2 weeks, the designated team member calls the patient and checks on their progress with the plan. The goal is to focus on taking the specific actions that have emerged and adjusting them using the SMART goals approach, moving the patient toward incremental success. SMART stands for goals that are specific, measurable, achievable, relevant, and time-based. SMART is a widely used, evidence-based approach to help people achieve behavior change and is a standard part of behavioral health and health coach training. See the American Institute for Cancer Research (AICR) guides to using SMART goals.[3]

Additional follow-up visits or calls with the team support member are scheduled every 2 to 4 weeks, or as appropriate. In the VA these visits or calls are called "touches." Often it takes up to 8 touches to establish a new behavior with patients.

The care path in Figure 11.3 is how we do it in our clinic, but there's no right or wrong way to engage patients in whole person care, as long as some time is spent addressing the person's health and healing needs. We have described the specifics here to show how one clinic operationalized the process. Many of the IOLC members already had established ways of expanding to whole person care. In those situations, they selected the tools and resources that fit their needs. In Chapter 15 we will describe approaches to help engage the team and leadership in making the practice changes needed to establish whole person care.

TIPS FOR DELIVERING WHOLE PERSON CARE

The primary care and oncology learning collaboratives that have used this approach have developed many tips for helping make whole person care successful. Some of the most salient suggestions are:

- Have a specific time set aside, either at a wellness visit, during infusions, or during survivorship visits, to discuss goals. This shows the team's commitment to whole person care.

- Prepare and display prominent descriptions about whole person care offered by the clinic.

- Have all tools, templates, and resources organized for easy use. Run educational seminars with the oncology team members on how to use them.

- Build the HOPE Note Toolkit items into the EHR to facilitate the process. The use of templates, dot phrases, and automatic coding processes is key.

- Use the PHI to guide the discussion and to streamline the visit.

- Use a listening, feedback, and summary process (sometimes called "teach back" as previously described) with the patient to help build trust and rapport.

- Send a follow-up summary of the PHP discussion to the patient.

- Focus on 1 to 3 identified areas. Try only a few changes at a time to increase the likelihood of success and continued behavior change. Other items can be put into a "parking lot" for future discussion, if needed.

- Ask how things are going with their life's meaning and purpose (what matters at the top of the PHI) at the beginning of follow-up visits; it is rewarding for patient and provider alike.

- Train staff in health coaching and patient advocacy; it is highly useful.

- Use a group visit strategy to efficiently and powerfully scale whole person care. One way to learn more about group visits for chronic illness and cancer is with training through the Integrative Center for Group Visit Training (www.icgmv.org).

- Adjust case conferences to allow time for discussion of a portion of the HOPE Note. This keeps whole person care embedded in the cancer treatment planning process.

- Dovetail these changes in practice for whole person care into the clinic or hospital's quality and practice improvement processes to routinize this care.

We encourage care teams to read the IOLC member case studies available on the Healing Works Foundation website for ideas on how to apply whole person care principles in oncology. In addition, Tufts University School of Medicine Office of Continuing Education provides a free 15-hour CME course on whole person care that takes learners step by step through practice change (www.IntegrativeHealthCME.org). While the course isn't focused on cancer care, the basic principles and steps for implementation are similar for all disciplines. A new, cancer-focused 3-hour course is in development as we write this book and should be completed by publication.

BUT I DON'T HAVE TIME

Care teams often say they do not have time to add person-centered care questions and management into a routine office visit. And that is true, the way most clinical flow processes are designed. But what really happens in the absence of a whole centered care process is that the actual time the care team spends with a patient is simply extended over many visits, calls, messages, made or missed appointments, and still patients' needs or questions may not seem (to them) to have been met. Patients may then wonder if they are getting the best care and, those who can, "shop around" looking for what might be nothing more than someone to listen and explain things. Once team members make the mental shift to whole person care and become used to routinely asking for "what matters" for the patient, addressing those needs becomes easier and faster.

Dr Jonas shares the story of how a telephonic HOPE visit made an impact:

> A 75-year-old man in a rural area called me 6 years into his treatment for an integrative consultation for bladder cancer that had spread despite local therapy. Obstruction from the cancer led eventually to external urinary diversion ("these damn tubes coming out of my back") which had limited his mobility. Living 3 hours from his oncologist and 4 hours from his daughter complicated his care. On the PHI he wrote that what mattered most to him was that his daughter not be burdened with his care and that he regain mobility to better care for himself. His daughter, he said, was to be married in 4 months and he wanted to be there. Surgical revisions of his tubes had been scheduled and twice cancelled. He was "fed up" and had lost trust in his doctors' ability to get him to that wedding.
>
> Listening, it became clear that his tumor treatment was appropriate to date (currently, immunotherapy), but his main goal was not being met. What he really needed was to transfer his care to a hospital closer to his daughter so as not to burden her with the long drives and where, if possible, surgical revision to improve his mobility would be easier to accomplish. This required a decision on his part to move (which he did with her help) and a "warm handoff" to a surgeon and oncologist to avoid any break in treatment. Now he was on track. The visit to discuss what mattered to him that the PHI had opened up took about 20 minutes.

TAKING THE NEXT STEPS

As Jenny Leyh said after learning how to care for herself and leading the Patient Advocacy and Empowerment Collaborative: "Empowering patients to self-advocate is key in the uptake of integrative modalities that will support healing and restore quality of life during cancer treatment and beyond."

In this chapter, we've provided resources and discussed how to use the HOPE Note Toolkit to provide whole person care. Note that the process is initiated by the oncology practice/team, not by the patients, so self-advocacy becomes less necessary and there is more time for healing. In Chapter 2, we described other ways to help patients self-advocate when such services aren't offered or available, and when what is needed or wanted differs from what is available.

We hope your team sees the inherent value in having patients activated in their care and an example of how one clinic uses an organized care pathway to make whole person care happen routinely. In cases when the patient doesn't want to or otherwise can't self-advocate, support for their wishes and monitoring for readiness is the best response. When you provide whole person cancer care, or signal to patients by offering HOPE visits that you believe their inherent self-knowledge and values are important aspects of their care, you are being a patient advocate. The next 2 chapters provide more details on the resources available to fully implement whole person care using this process. We start with the most important activities: tools for self-care that anyone can do.

SUMMARY POINTS

- Making whole person care routine and regular requires having the tools, training, and resources available to deliver it in the flow of clinical practice.

- Tools and resources to do this were adapted from primary care by the Integrative Oncology Leadership Collaborative (IOLC) and the Patient Advocacy and Empowerment Collaborative (PAEC). They are collectively called the HOPE

Note Toolkit and are designed to help make whole person cancer care easier.

- The central tool in that toolkit is the Personal Health Inventory (PHI), a patient-facing form designed to communicate what whole person care is and assess what matters most to a person.

- Time is needed to have these discussions with patients; the amount of time is manageable and may prevent wasted time and energy in future episodic care.

- PHI review can be done in a separate visit or done with focus in one of the standard planning visits.

CHAPTER TWELVE

OPTIMIZING SELF-CARE

Self-care behaviors are the key for creating a tumor microenvironment (TME) favorable to controlling cancer and optimizing quality and length of life. Some people have been following these practices (or at least some of them) since they were children. Some have never learned how to incorporate them into their daily habits. Regardless of where the person starts, oncology teams providing whole person care should offer to help patients enhance their self-care activities. In addition to helping people feel better, this support, when done well, can empower patients to take more control of their health and life in general, which is an important characteristic of recovery. In Chapter 4 we reviewed the core wellness factors for health optimization and the evidence for their benefits in those with cancer. In this chapter, we will discuss the process of behavior change and provide a set of practical resources and tools care teams can use with patients to help them incorporate self-care more fully.

CHANGING BEHAVIOR

Oncology teams often get discouraged about changing patient behavior. Many of us have known people who continue to smoke, for example, even after getting lung cancer. However, this pessimism primarily arises because teams have not been taught how to use the extensive science of behavior change, nor have they designed their care processes and trained their teams to use that science. When we use science-based techniques to encourage behavior change, we often see the change happen.

Unlike the way medicine is often practiced, where the doctor tells the patient what to do and then judges their adherence, behavior change involves partnering between the care team and the person to develop specific, incremental goals, and then collaborating with them to implement those changes, one (sometimes slow) step at a time. When this happens, we feel good about our ability to support changes toward self-care and wellness, while patients feel good about their ability to make other changes in their life toward self-care and wellness.

Be the Behavior You Want to See

Creating wellbeing in others starts with creating wellbeing in oneself—healing the healer. The tools we describe in this chapter are designed for use with patients, but the first step for any team moving toward whole person care is to offer them to the clinical team members themselves.

Questions for the team include, "What can I do to support my own healing through self-care and behavior change? How can my own health journey help me lead people facing cancer to new levels of health and healing? What are the foundational tenets of healing and wellbeing? How do I embed them in my life? How can our clinic create a culture of health and make self-care and wellbeing a priority?" One robust way teams can ask and start to answer these questions is to make key elements of self-care into a month-long theme, perhaps including a 1-hour workshop, lunch and learn, or grand rounds. Start with these topics:

- Environment/healing spaces
- Activity (movement/exercise, yoga, tai chi)
- Nutrition

- Sleep

- Stress management

- Social and emotional support

- Mental and spiritual support

- Herbs and supplements

HEALING SPACES: OPTIMIZING THE ENVIRONMENT

We can think about the physical environment as the surroundings, conditions, circumstances, or objects in and around where we live and operate. Making the spaces where you live, work, and play into healing spaces can reduce triggers that may cause stress and impact health.

By incorporating elements of evidence-based design into a physical space, the space can become a healing place for relaxing, resting, and recharging.

1. Surround yourself with nature or views of nature.

2. Decorate with meaning and purpose. Personal items and how furniture is arranged can encourage interaction and conversation.

3. Simplify the space. Declutter.

4. Choose colors thoughtfully. To energize and stimulate, choose shades of yellow, red, and orange; to calm and evoke rest, choose shades of violet, blue, and green.

5. Ensure the bedroom is dark and clutter-free for optimal sleep.

Encourage patients to connect with nature, as the outdoors can be a powerful healing space. Physical benefits of exposure to nature include:

- Lower stress hormone levels

- Reduced resting heart rate

- Improved mood

- Fewer depressive symptoms

- Boosted natural killer cells in the body that are important for fighting infection and cancer

Trees, for instance, emit healing essential oils called phytoncides that have a positive impact on immune cells.[1] Stepping outside for fresh air, visiting a forest (forest bathing), or just sitting by a window and looking out at the sky, grass, or trees can make an impact. One study showed that surgery patients who had a room looking out on nature were discharged a full day earlier than those that looked at a brick wall.[2]

PHYSICAL ACTIVITY

"You need to rest" is outdated guidance for most people with cancer—in fact, it can even be harmful advice. Study after study shows that physical movement boosts the immune system, relieves anxiety, improves fatigue, improves cardiopulmonary function,[3] increases pain tolerance, and builds strength and flexibility,[4] whether the person is in cancer treatment or is aiming to boost their health as a survivor. Properly used, exercise at the appropriate level is not only safe and beneficial for people with cancer but can also help prevent recurrence.

Additionally, physical activity also has mental and quality-of-life benefits.[5] It can help provide a greater sense of control for people dealing with the uncertainties of cancer.[6] Oncologists can consider an "exercise prescription," especially for those who would benefit from physical therapy or who are recovering from surgery and need medical supervision.

Personalized movement plans are beneficial both for those in treatment and as survivors. The American College of Sports Medicine (ACSM) recommends some level of physical activity for *all* cancer survivors.[7] We know that just 30 minutes of moderate-intensity movement, such as walking 3 times a week, can significantly reduce cancer risk.

When working with a person to increase their activity level, encourage them to think of it as something enjoyable and beneficial, not an unpleasant chore. Movement includes any activity, such as:

- Walking or hiking
- Participation in active sports such as tennis, soccer, or basketball
- A workout at a gym
- Recreational activities such as dancing, bicycling, swimming, skiing, fishing, or martial arts
- Group aerobic activities such as step class or Zumba®
- Active gardening, yard work, or housework
- Movement therapies such as yoga, qigong, and tai chi
- Chair exercises, resistance bands, and water aerobics for people who have limited mobility or strength

Finding an activity that's *fun* will increase motivation, enjoyment, and the chance that a person will do it on an ongoing basis, even after cancer treatment is over. Movement can also be combined with social activities, strengthening connections to family and friends, and increasing motivation.

Helping people to increase physical movement works better when we take a health coaching approach to behavior change. Encourage people to pursue activities that interest them and explore new ones. Align their interests and abilities with resources available online, in the clinic, or in the community. Inexpensive coaches and groups are available in many community centers and through organizations such as the YMCA, Boys and Girls Clubs, and local community and recreation centers. Most Medicare Advantage plans offer members 65 and older free in person and online gym memberships through the Silver Sneakers Program®. Many other low cost and free options are available locally and regionally. Several of the Integrative Oncology Leadership Council (IOLC) sites make movement classes—in person and online—free for patients, family members and the community. The nonprofit Karuna Precision Wellness Center in Indianapolis, for example, offers low cost and free online movement classes and personal training options oriented to people with cancer.

The ACSM provides a downloadable guide to exercise, including recommendations for specific cancer symptoms and treatment side effects.[8] The Maple Tree Cancer Alliance (www.mapletreecanceralliance.org) provides individualized exercise programs—both in person and virtually—to help relieve some of the side effects related to cancer treatment. Virtual memberships are very inexpensive; they also provide clinical exercise programs that hospitals can offer to patients.

NUTRITION

The question, "What should l eat?" is very common after a cancer diagnosis. It may be prompted by concern for maintaining strength or coping with side effects, or even by the search for a cancer-curing diet.

"Whatever you feel like eating—it doesn't really matter" is often the unproductive answer. Oncologists see many patients lose their appetites, struggle with nausea, and lose or gain unwanted weight during treatment. However, they receive little training in nutrition to manage these concerns.[9]

Nutrition consultation is the most reported (35%) complementary therapy used by patients during cancer treatment.[10] Oncology dieticians or nutritionists are an important part of the care team to work not only with the patient, but their caregivers as well, to teach them about healthy eating and any special dietary needs the person with cancer may have during treatment. Social workers can also be brought in to help patients qualify for Meals on Wheels programs or other meal delivery services.

Healthy eating is generally accepted as an important part of cancer treatment. According to the ACS, healthy eating can help a person:

- Feel better during and after treatment
- Stay stronger and more energetic

- Maintain a healthy weight
- Give the body key calories and nutrients
- Better tolerate side effects from treatment
- Lower infection risk
- Heal and recover faster

A personalized approach is key, as food does more than just fuel us physically. It's loaded with meaning and emotion. Food is family, culture, tradition, and comfort. It can even be used to self-medicate. Knowing why a person chooses the foods they eat is critical.

Research shows many connections between diet and cancer, from the strong association of cancer risk with factors such as obesity, alcohol consumption, and processed meat,[11] to the potential benefits of a diet high in carotene- and sulforaphane-containing foods, such as broccoli.[12]

Deciding what and how to eat during and beyond treatment means using common sense amid conflicting and confusing messages from the many unqualified "experts" found online. Recommendations range from fasting and eliminating all animal food to a low-carbohydrate, high-fat (ketogenic) diet. Few of the recommendations are truly evidence based. So far, only a Mediterranean-like diet has been proven to reduce the risk of cancer.[13] The impact of this simple change can be profound. A large, randomized controlled trial for example showed that eating a Mediterranean diet with additional nuts added reduced the incidence of breast cancer by 47%.[14] A good resource for patients is the Mediterranean Diet Pocket Guide, available from the Healing Works Foundation.

Food can help heal the body, mind, and spirit. It can convey the message "I care about you" from a caregiver and help people with cancer focus on self-care. Often, a medical diagnosis such as cancer is an inflection point for a person and their family to move to a healthier diet as part of healing and survivorship. Foods that fight cancer and inflammation contribute to whole person healing regardless of the ultimate treatment outcome. These include dark-green and deep-yellow vegetables, citrus fruits, whole grains, nuts, and legumes. Rebecca Katz's cookbook *The Cancer-Fighting Kitchen* is a great resource for patients to create healing and delicious foods.[15] Additional resources are available from the Smith Center for Healing and the Arts in Washington, DC (www.smith-center.org). For an in-depth discussion of nutrition for people with cancer, check Nutrition in Cancer Care Physician Data Query (PDQ) from the NCI.[16] PDQ here is not to be confused with the Patient Dignity Question, found on page 2 of the Personal Health Inventory (PHI). For additional information on healthy eating, look to your local community. Many community hospitals offer free talks and classes, for example.

When treatment affects the person's ability to eat, the oncology team should arrange for a consultation with a nutritionist. Mouth sores, mucositis, nausea, reduced appetite, weight gain or loss, and other treatment side effects can lead to malnutrition and dehydration, with serious consequences. Nutritionists can also help with anorexia and cachexia, and overeating.

HERBS AND SUPPLEMENTS

Most people with cancer take supplements, including vitamins, minerals, herbs, and other substances, before, during, or after their treatment. Because information about many of these supplements is often confusing and based on inadequate evidence, oncology teams might be tempted to tell people with cancer to just stop taking them out of concern for drug interactions. However, some supplements—both ones to consider and to avoid—are supported by evidence. This is a growing area of research, with new evidence emerging frequently. See Chapter 5 for a list of the best information sources for supplements and cancer.

Because supplement use is so common, patients should be asked specifically about which, if any, they take. This should be done while asking about current prescription and over-the-counter medications. The questions could be, "Do you take any herbs or supplements? If so, which ones and how much?"

A 2014 study showed a more complete version of the question is: "Do you use any natural, folk, traditional, grandma remedies, herbs picked in the garden, infusions, or herbal teas to improve your health?"[17] This question makes clear that you are asking about *all* supplements, not just the usual vitamins, minerals, and common herbs.

Many patients don't disclose this information to their care team for fear of being judged or told to stop the supplement, so it's important to show an open mind and willingness to discuss. Being sensitive to the cultural importance of folk and traditional remedies can increase communication. You can ask whether the family values any traditional practices, such as traditional Chinese medicine or Ayurvedic medicine.

The top supplements to *avoid* are:

- St. John's wort. Decreases efficacy of chemotherapy drugs and has many drug interactions; increases skin problems from radiation.

- Acetyl-L-carnitine (ALC). Worsens nerve damage from chemotherapy. Previously, it was thought to help with this.

- Vitamin E. Patients who took vitamin E while smoking during treatment for head and neck cancers had higher rates of recurrence and eventual death.[18] Vitamin E can also increase the risk of prostate cancer.[19]

- Beta-carotene. In a large study, beta-carotene increased the risk of lung cancer in men who smoked.

Using supplements as part of whole person cancer care means using them in 3 ways:

1. Using supplements in cases of nutrient depletion from drug side effects

2. Monitoring safe use of supplements patients are already taking

3. Recommending supplements therapeutically as treatments for side effects

For a list of safer supplements for cancer and treatment, see the Supplements and Cancer Pocket Guide from the Healing Works Foundation. The guide covers the most commonly used supplements, including ginger, ginseng, probiotics, coenzyme Q10 (coQ10), vitamin B12, vitamin C, zinc, melatonin, and others.

Remind patients to purchase only quality supplements from reputable brands. Look for the NSF International, US Pharmacopeia, or Consumer Lab seal on the label. These organizations verify what's inside the product. Certification can also help ensure the supplements aren't contaminated by pesticides, heavy metals, or other dangerous substances and that the products are of high quality and accurately labeled.

Useful databases or sources for clinicians to find quality information on supplements include:

- US Pharmacopoeia information on dietary supplements and food at Dietary Supplements | Quality Matters | U.S. Pharmacopeia Blog (usp.org)
- Dietary and Herbal Supplements Guide at the National Center for Complementary and Integrative Health
- ConsumerLab.com (paid subscription) for reviews of supplements and other health products
- FDA Dietary Supplement Ingredient Advisory List; sign up to get alerts when new ingredients are added. The FDA's What's New in Dietary Supplements page has the latest news and actions.
- Physician Data Query (PDQ) from the NCI
- About Herbs from Memorial Sloan Kettering Cancer Center (MSKCC)
- Natural Medicines database
- Wellkasa (commercial site) for science on supplements and information on drug-supplement interactions
- CancerChoices website supplements information
- KNOW Database on natural products studied in cancer

SLEEP AND CANCER

Studies suggest that 59% of people with cancer experience disordered sleep, as compared to estimates of 10 to 30% among the cancer-free American population.[20] Improved sleep may be the strongest foundation a person can build to support healing. Ask people about their sleep at every appointment. If they're not sleeping well, you need to know so that the care team can address their concerns. Ask patients with poor sleep to consider keeping a journal for middle-of-the-night thoughts so that they can bring up any cancer-related items at their next appointment or in counseling.

Both cancer treatment itself and the worries related to having cancer can negatively impact sleep. Cancer treatment commonly includes the use of steroids (for example, dexamethasone or prednisone), which directly impair sleep quality and may cause insomnia. Additionally, sleep-disrupting treatment side effects like hot flashes, which occur in both men and women, and cancer-related fatigue, including from postsurgical pain or neuropathy, make sleep quantity and quality even more important.

In addition to standard sleep hygiene guidance and pharmaceutical interventions, nondrug approaches like exercise, guided meditation, and mindfulness meditation should be considered. Strong evidence supports exercise and cognitive behavioral therapy (CBT-I) for insomnia. Any modality that supports whole person healing and is of interest to the patient may be explored. These may include yoga, tai chi, acupuncture, light therapy, cannabis, or supplements of the hormone melatonin, which helps regulate circadian (day/night) rhythm (When using melatonin, choose a high-quality product from a reputable source.).

Light therapy exposes you to bright light similar to natural sunlight as a way to restore your natural circadian (day/night) rhythm. It can be helpful for sleep disorders, especially if they are caused by lack of exposure to natural light or if your normal sleep pattern has been disrupted by hospitalization.[21] Some evidence suggests that blue light from LEDs and screens (TVs, computers, phones) before bedtime can disrupt sleep by reducing your production of melatonin so you don't fall asleep quickly.[22] If this is a problem, avoiding blue light for 2 to 3 hours before bedtime may help. Glasses that block blue light may also be helpful.

Many patients report using cannabis, THC, or CBD to help them relax or sleep, but there is currently little data on cannabis use for sleep in cancer.[23] Some data suggests tumor response to immunotherapy may be blunted in those using cannabis. [24] Laws on cannabis use vary from state to state and are in constant flux. In states where it's prohibited, people with cancer may be using it for sleep and not telling their doctors.

A good source for more information about sleep and cancer is CancerChoices' sleep page. The Integrative Approaches for Better Sleep Pocket Guide from the Healing Works Foundation is a good reference to give patients. For a high-quality sleep measurement tool, use the Pittsburgh Sleep Quality Index (PSQI). This self-rated questionnaire evaluates overall sleep quality over a 1-month time interval by using nineteen self-reported items to assess sleep quality and disturbances.

STRESS AND DISTRESS MANAGEMENT

We all experience stress, but for those who currently have or have gone through cancer or other serious illnesses, stress is both an acute and chronic presence. It tends to flare up around procedures, tests, and treatment and lingers long after. As cancer survivor Jenny Leyh found, the stresses of daily life intensified after her diagnosis and escalated in the year after chemotherapy ended. Even though she had been declared "no evidence of disease," the thought of recurrence was always in the back of her mind. To deal with the stress and anxiety this caused, she turned to a combination of antidepressants, yoga, meditation, and cannabis, eventually finding the mix that worked for her. Each patient requires their own recipe for managing the unavoidable stress of cancer diagnosis, treatment, and life after cancer.

Sometimes, such as during cancer treatment, reducing stress just isn't possible. In these times, patients need understanding and support from their medical team and caregivers. This is also when encouraging people to learn how to engage the relaxation response and mindfulness pays off in better resilience. When people can call on the relaxation response to quiet the mind and use mindfulness to distance their thoughts, stress processes are reduced.

Helping patients develop their own recipe for reducing stress can be very helpful for healing. A useful assessment tool is the FACT GP (Functional Assessment of Cancer Therapy-General Population), which measures emotional distress tolerance in a 21-item instrument that assesses physical, social/family, emotional, and functional well-being. A shortened, 7-item version, FACT-G7, is designed to capture the most relevant issues quickly and effectively. The Edmonton Symptom Assessment System (ESAS-r) is also a short and widely used and validated tool for tracking common symptoms in people with advanced cancer. Whatever measures or patient-reported outcomes your clinic uses, the important thing is to respond to what the inquiry finds.

Journaling

Journaling, also known as therapeutic writing, can help people with cancer identify and manage emotional distress and other issues, both during and after treatment. Journaling or writing has been found in many studies to reduce feelings of depression, anxiety, and stress that can come when facing the challenge of cancer.[25] Journaling can help patients express thought patterns, such as identity concerns, and emotions such as fear, anger, sadness, and helplessness. Journaling about these feelings helps people learn to tolerate them and helps them resist catastrophic thinking and think more rationally. Expressing thoughts on paper (or screen) helps reframe thinking and deescalates emotional responses.

Journaling is helpful for managing social and emotional needs. Good questions for people to explore include: What does support mean to you? What has support looked like for you in the past? Who is in your current support network? This self-reflection offers an opportunity for people to identify and tap into resources and to better understand their own needs and beliefs. A journal is also a safe, private place to express thoughts and emotions that might be distressing for caregivers and others to hear.

A gratitude journal, kept as part of journaling or instead of it, can be another helpful tool. Listing several things, no matter how trivial, to be grateful for each day can help people gain perspective on their life with cancer.[26]

For patients who are anxious, having difficulty sleeping, or are reluctant to express their emotions to others, journaling is a beneficial, safe, free technique that involves no drugs or interventions. Patients can use their journal to write down any questions or observations they want to bring to the care team's attention. It is an easy way to help empower them if suggested as a "healing assignment" between visits.

SOCIAL AND EMOTIONAL SUPPORT: COPING WITH THE TRAUMA OF CANCER

A cancer diagnosis can lead to cancer-related post-traumatic stress, both from the diagnostic label itself and from the treatment. The NCI defines cancer-related post-traumatic stress as "A condition that develops in some people who are diagnosed with cancer. Symptoms of cancer-related post-traumatic stress (PTS) include having frightening thoughts or trouble sleeping, being distracted or overexcited, feeling alone, or losing interest in daily activities. Symptoms may also include feelings of shock, fear, helplessness, or horror. Crucially, the NCI points out, "Cancer-related PTS can occur any time after diagnosis, including during or after treatment." Cancer patients deal with their disease every day for months, years, and even the rest of their lives. The cumulative effect can tip over to PTS at any point. Oncology team members need to be alert to signs of cancer-related PTS, even in people who seem to be handling the situation well.

Modalities such as yoga and mind-body techniques can be helpful for stress reduction, but PTS goes beyond ordinary cancer stress. Patients may need more direct help, including medication or referral to a mental health provider.[27] A valuable source for thinking about trauma and how to treat it is *Transforming Trauma: The Path to Hope and Healing,* by James S. Gordon, MD.[28]

The Importance of Social Support

Social support is an evidence-based aspect of mainstream cancer care. Social and professional interactions that foster a sense of belonging, wellbeing, and coherence are healing relationships. Nurturing healing relationships are one of the most powerful ways to stimulate, support, and maintain wellness and recovery.

Social support is emotional support, practical help, and advice. Common types of social support are:

- Informal support and practical help from family and friends
- Support groups
- Individual counseling
- Online communities
- Tools to communicate with family and friends, such as CaringBridge

Oncology teams see many people who have great support from family and friends—and they also see people who are facing their diagnosis entirely alone. Not surprisingly, those solo patients often don't do as well physically or mentally—and even those with plenty of support sometimes need additional help. Even with good social support, conflict or tension may arise between the patient and family members; providing social work or chaplain support or counseling for the family can help during those times.

Support Groups

Cancer support groups can provide people with encouragement, comfort, and advice. They are an accepted and valuable part of care. Groups help those with similar situations share their experience and concerns with each other, express feelings others might not understand, and learn more about how to cope. Importantly, they can help people feel less alone. This can help all people with cancer, but it is particularly helpful for people in minority racial or ethnic groups or those with rare cancers, such as men with breast cancer or young people with cancer. They have specific needs even other cancer patients might not understand, making them feel isolated. Support groups can provide these people with much-needed encouragement, advice, and information.

In person support groups for people with cancer are often organized by local hospitals and community organizations. The group is generally led by a social worker, psychologist, trained patient advocate, or other professional. Advocacy associations such as the ACS, the Colon Cancer Alliance, and the National Breast Cancer Foundation can help people connect with local support groups. The social worker on the oncology team or at a local hospital is usually the best source of information about support groups. Group visits within the clinical setting can also function as support groups. (To learn more about implementing group visits, check the Integrated Center for Group Medical Visits at www.icgmv.org.)

Support groups are also available online. This is a good option when there's no local group and may actually be preferable for people who have transportation limitations or are too debilitated by treatment to attend in-person meetings. To find these, check with advocacy associations and ask the social worker.

Patient Advocates

Patient advocates are personal guides who help people get the right care at the right time during their cancer journey. They can take the form of a friend or family member, a social worker, nurse navigator, or a former cancer patient—and the person with cancer, who is their own best advocate. A patient advocate can assist with the practical aspects of cancer treatment, such as helping someone find ways to pay for treatment and living expenses, access health insurance, get transportation to appointments, access to community resources, housing, and more.

A family member or friend who knows the patient well can join them at appointments to support and advocate for them. They can let the care team know about things the patient might not mention, such as symptoms and mental outlook. They can be a connecting bridge for the care team, providing crucial information.

Cancer centers and hospitals have professional patient advocates, sometimes called patient navigators or health care advocates. If your cancer center doesn't assign a patient navigator or advocate to a person in your practice, ask for one. If none is available, the care team can help by putting people in touch with local and national nonprofit organizations, federally qualified health centers, government agencies, insurance companies, and for-profit patient advocacy firms. A resource list for patient navigation, case management, and patient advocates can be found in the Pocket Guide to Patient Advocacy in Cancer on the Healing Works Foundation website.

SPIRITUALITY

When we talk about spiritual life, we usually mean a connection to something beyond ourselves—the higher power that 90% of Americans believe in. You can be spiritual whether or not you are also religious, belong to a faith group, or follow specific principles and beliefs. Spirituality and religion both help us answer the big questions of existence: Why am I here? What is the meaning of life? What matters? Self-transcendence is often the goal and is at the top of Maslow's revised hierarchy of needs as shown in Chapter 1.

Cancer and other serious illnesses tend to draw our attention to these questions. Many studies show that having a spiritual or religious practice helps people with cancer cope with challenges ranging from depression and anxiety to pain management and recovery.[29] According to the 2022 survey US Patient & Oncologist Awareness, Usage, & Attitudes Toward Whole Person Integrative Oncology, spiritual services are in the top five complementary therapies used during treatment, used by at least 25% of patients.[30]

Cancer and its management can raise needs a person was unaware of before. Raymond Wadlow, MD, a medical oncologist at the Inova Schar Cancer Care Center in Fairfax, Virginia, says common questions include:

- Why me?

- Is cancer my fault?

- Is God or the universe punishing or testing me?

- Did this happen because I smoked, drank alcohol, ate certain foods, or did something bad in the past?

- Will I die soon?

- What will happen to my spirit after I die?

- Has my life mattered?

Worrying about these questions—spiritual distress—can have a negative effect on the person's physical, social, and emotional quality of life. On the other hand, spiritual care has been found to positively impact quality of life[31] and can be especially helpful at the end of life.[32] Even if a person isn't religious, it can still be important to discuss their fears, worries, and questions.

Chaplains

Although many patients say they want to discuss spiritual issues,[33] members of the cancer care team may be hesitant to bring up spiritual life because they don't want to intrude on personal beliefs. Many may feel they don't have the expertise to discuss spiritual or religious issues with patients. Some are uncomfortable discussing these issues or believe discussing them is unethical. This is where a chaplain can help. The doctor asks, "What's the matter?" but the chaplain asks, "What matters?"

A chaplain is a trained spiritual leader who works at a hospital or for another organization such as a branch of the military service, work site, school or community organization. Most service members are familiar with chaplains, who may come from any faith and are generally trained to help people of all faiths or none.

Your hospital or cancer center probably has one or more chaplains who can provide spiritual support and pastoral care for patients and family members. They can talk with patients about spiritual concerns and health care decisions. Just as importantly, they can support members of the care team at the hospital or clinic.[34]

Social workers and therapists, including art and music therapists, can also help patients deal with challenging questions about spirituality and cancer. Patients can also be encouraged to reconnect with their spiritual community, even if they have not been active recently—or ever.

A spiritual assessment tool can help honor and accommodate a person's belief system and spiritual practices. One widely used tool is the FICA Spiritual History Tool. (The acronym stands for F: faith and beliefs, I: importance of spirituality in your life, C: spiritual community of support, and A: how does the patient wish these addressed.) The tool is a guide for clinicians to incorporate open-ended questions regarding spirituality into a standard comprehensive history and determine when referral to a chaplain is appropriate.[35] If the Personal Health Inventory (PHI) used during a HOPE visit identifies spiritual and religious areas as important to the patient, use of the FICA or asking if they would like to see a chaplain can be a next step.

To learn more about the connection between medicine and spirituality, read *Healing Words: The Power of Prayer and the Practice of Medicine* by Larry Dossey, MD. Dr Dossey explores the link between medicine and spirituality, and he concludes that prayer and spirituality are a critical part of a person's ability to heal.[36]

SUMMARY POINTS

- Self-care behaviors are at the core of optimizing whole person cancer care.

- There is a robust science of behavior change. Teams can become effective in behavior change by getting training in and using that science.

- We summarize the key resources available to assist in self-care in the key areas of the physical environment, activity, nutrition, herbs and supplements, stress management, social support, sleep and spirituality.

- Picking up one or more of these areas as topics for training and team development is the best way to start bringing them into routine care.

CHAPTER THIRTEEN

SUPPORTIVE AND INTEGRATIVE SERVICES

Supportive and integrative services in cancer care have slowly been increasing in evidence and use over several decades. Advances in immune therapy and our understanding of the importance of the tumor microenvironment (TME) and now macroenvironment in cancer has now further solidified the value of these areas in whole person care. The history of alternative and complementary medicine and its integration into mainstream medicine has been fraught with controversy and a gradual sorting out of the wheat from the chaff. Clarity is emerging.

For decades, anything not designed to kill the cancer cells was labeled "quackery," "unconventional," or "alternative," and was largely shunned by oncologists, researchers, regulators, and insurers. Patients with cancer, on the other hand, often sought out and used such practices, usually without good evidence or guidance and at their own risk. Many patients would not discuss these practices with their doctors, further widening the communication and risk gap. Slowly, evidence accumulated showing benefit from some of these practices. Many of them were already being used in supportive and palliative care. Many were allowed or even incorporated into mainstream care, becoming first "complementary" and then "integrative." Some services, such as nutrition for overall health and mind-body practices for mental health support, lost their alternative label and became fully available and even recommended as standard of care. Others, such as yoga and acupuncture, have become available in a spottier fashion, and retain the name "complementary" or, when merged into routine oncology, "integrative."

These practices continue to evolve as knowledge about them and a deeper understanding of how they influence the TME, and the person as a whole, emerges. The overlap and alliance with supportive care, palliative care, patient-centered care, and other areas has become more evident.

The key questions for the team are: What can my patients safely tap into using non-drug approaches and from complementary and alternative medicine? How do I make sure they don't harm themselves by pursuing such therapies? How do I help them find and recommend modalities they can afford? What, if anything, is covered by insurance? Where are the best places for me to learn about these modalities? How can I teach patients about these when I don't have time to do integrative oncology training myself?

In the last chapter we provided information and resources to use with patients and the team for self-care. In this chapter, we describe the most prominent supportive and integrative practices and services delivered by professionals and point to resources and how teams can use these services as part of routine care.

• • •

What follows are short descriptions of several supportive and integrative services that can be provided for patients. We will also point oncology teams toward places where these services are available if the team doesn't have them in their clinic or system. Many of these services are scattered, making them difficult to access and coordinate. Organizing them into a single delivery system, as in the Two-Circle Model or an integrative practice unit as described in Chapter 15, can streamline their access and delivery.

ACUPRESSURE AND ACUPUNCTURE

The 2022 SIO-ASCO guidelines recommend acupuncture and acupressure for general cancer or musculoskeletal pain.

Acupressure

Acupressure stimulates energy flow throughout your body and many people say their energy increases after an acupressure or acupuncture session. Traditional Chinese medicine teaches that energy (qi) flows through pathways (meridians) in the body. To rebalance energy, hands and fingers or a special device are used to put pressure on specific points along the pathways. A therapist can do acupressure, but it is also easy to self-teach online. A person with cancer can learn to do it for themselves; people in their support network can also learn how to do it.

According to the SIO, people with cancer use acupressure for fatigue, nausea, and vomiting from chemotherapy, pain, and stress.

Acupuncture

Like acupressure, acupuncture is part of traditional Chinese medicine. To rebalance energy, very thin acupuncture needles are inserted into specific points along these pathways. According to Chinese medicine theory, this engages healing by stimulating and balancing energy flow throughout the body. Western explanations of acupuncture mechanisms have also been studied, such as induction of endogenous opioids and stimulation of the autonomic system.[1] Acupuncture is usually done with needles, but it can also be done with mild electrical stimulation, or light (usually cold lasers) instead. This is sometimes called acustimulation or electroacupuncture.

Acupuncture treatment is provided by acupuncturists, medical doctors, nurses, and other trained health care providers. In most states, acupuncturists must be certified by the National Certification Commission for Acupuncture and Oriental Medicine (NCCAOM). Some states don't require certification, but limit which providers can do acupuncture. Nearly all states require licensure.

Acupuncture has been shown to decrease pain and mitigate nausea and vomiting from chemotherapy. Solid studies show that acupuncture can reduce joint pain in women with early-stage hormone positive breast cancer who are taking aromatase inhibitors. In one randomized clinical trial published in *JAMA,* for example, women with aromatase inhibitor-related joint pain had reduced pain both in the short term (after 6 weeks of acupuncture) and long term (after 52 weeks) compared with controls, suggesting long-term benefits of this therapy. In particular, acupuncture may help women on aromatase inhibitor therapy manage the side effect of joint pain so they can continue with the drug.[2]

Acupuncture is often used for anxiety and stress, fatigue, hot flashes, mood problems, and depression. The military (and VA) uses a form of acupuncture for pain and PTSD.[3] Both Jan and Jenny regularly use (and recommend) acupuncture both during active treatment and afterward.

AROMATHERAPY

Aromatherapy has a long history as an intervention that can improve an array of symptoms. It is the therapeutic use of essential oils (also known as volatile oils) from plants (flowers, herbs, or trees) for the improvement of physical, emotional, and spiritual wellbeing. In the US and UK, nurses have carried out much of the research on aromatherapy for symptom management in oncology. There is data for use of aromatherapy to prevent nausea, lessen anxiety, and improve sleep. For more information on this topic, see the NIH PDQ on aromatherapy. It is one of a dozen complementary and alternative therapy PDQ topics updated regularly, and can be found in a format for health professionals (https://www.cancer. gov/about-cancer/treatment/cam/hp/aromatherapy-pdq) and in one for patients (https://www.cancer.gov/about-cancer/treatment/ cam/patient/aromatherapy-pdq).

ART THERAPY

Art therapy is a form of clinical intervention that uses art as the primary mode of expression and communication. The art therapist uses creativity to help achieve personal and treatment-related goals. The patient makes and uses art to convey feelings at that moment or to dive deeper into a particular experience or situation. Art therapy has been found to have a positive impact on physical and psychological symptoms relating to cancer.[4]

When people are experiencing intense, complex, or confusing emotions, the use of art in a therapeutic setting can help them manage and communicate their feelings in ways that language can't always accomplish. You don't have to be "good" at art or an experienced artist to enjoy the benefits of art therapy. Jan at first resisted art therapy when an artist in residence came into the chemotherapy infusion room where she was getting treatment. After making a remarkable collage that gave her insight into some of the struggles she was having, she was sold on it and now does art classes at the local art center in her town. The adage "Try it, you'll like it" seems to apply to many of these practices.

Art therapy is widely considered a safe way of addressing physical and mental conditions when delivered by a well-trained and certified art therapist. Any form of therapy can unearth uncomfortable emotions and may cause you to experience increased levels of psychological discomfort. Reliving traumatic experiences is difficult. If it isn't handled correctly, it can negatively impact an individual's psychological and/or physical health. Psychological support from someone trained to give it may be needed. Still, this is no reason not to implement art therapy. Sometimes healing is hard.

If a person with cancer expresses interest in art therapy, guide them to the American Art Therapy Association which oversees and certifies the registration of art therapists and has a directory to locate qualified practitioners. Despite the evidence for its value, art therapy isn't usually covered by health insurance. The INOVA Health System (a member of the IOLC) provides art therapy to all its patients and family members free of charge.

MUSIC THERAPY

Music therapy is a well-recognized clinical intervention that uses music within a therapeutic process to assist the patient in identifying and dealing with social, cognitive, emotional, or physical concerns, including pain and fatigue. It's effective[5] for a number of mental health conditions and pain, and noninvasive, without risk of side effects.

A trained music therapist tailors the intervention to the individual's needs and helps them achieve therapeutic goals. The musical intervention may involve music coming from the therapist. Or it may involve the patient playing a musical instrument, singing, composing music, listening to, or dancing/moving to a piece of music. Music therapy allows the patient to express feelings or thoughts in a more complex and multidimensional manner than with words only and can help the patient address traumatic or uncomfortable situations without the use of words.

Cancer patients who participated in music therapy were better able to manage their symptoms, expressed more hope about their ability to survive cancer, and were better able to access and discuss traumatic memories associated with their diagnosis.[6] Music therapy has also been shown to decrease stress, anxiety, and depression in cancer patients, as well as have a small effect on fatigue.[7] The 2022 SIO-ASCO joint guideline for pain recommend music therapy for patients experiencing surgical pain.

Music medicine is also available to help alleviate general patient suffering. It involves patients listening to pre-recorded music offered by the medical team, rather than a trained music therapist. This provides a low- to no-cost option and may generate community between your team and patients that would not otherwise occur without music, the universal language. When patients are admitted to the hospital for pain control, Dr Jonas routinely recommends and offers music therapy as an adjunct to the usual pain treatments used.

The website of the American Music Therapy Association (www.musictherapy.org) allows you to search by therapist, certification, and the condition you would like to treat. The Certification Board for Music Therapists (www.cbmt.org) also offers a search feature.

FINANCIAL SUPPORT SERVICES

Cancer and its treatment can have serious, sometimes lasting effects on a person's finances. In one large survey, approximately 4 in 10 people with cancer said their out-of-pocket expenses (self-paid) were higher than they expected.[8]

The costs of cancer include much more than treatment. Unpaid sick time, loss of income from being unable to work, loss of income for caregivers, insurance copays, losing health insurance, medications, transportation, parking, medications, and a myriad of other unexpected expenses (childcare, for example) can accumulate to cause financial toxicity—problems related to the cost of medical care that may lead to debt and bankruptcy. People with cancer are 2.5 times more likely to file for bankruptcy than those without cancer; the mortality rate for those who do file for bankruptcy is 80% higher than those who don't file for bankruptcy.[9] Financial toxicity also affects quality of life and access to medical care. People with cancer experiencing financial toxicity may not fill prescriptions and may skip medical appointments, with serious consequences for their health and wellbeing.

Coping with Financial Toxicity

When the latest chemotherapy drug or treatment is extremely expensive, it "creates a lot of anxiety," says Raymond Wadlow, MD, a medical oncologist at the Inova Schar Cancer Center Institute in Fairfax, Virginia. His approach? Talking about financial options with every person who needs treatment, without guessing who might face financial challenges. "I simply say, 'We could do this treatment, or here are some other less costly options.'" This can help start a discussion about which treatment is the best choice overall.

"Doctors don't know much about financial toxicity, and patients often don't tell them much," Dr Wadlow says. "People may be apprehensive about sharing financial concerns with the cancer care team because they are wary of having the "budget" option recommended. They want to hear about the best care, not the lowest-cost option, because that may seem like it's less effective." This is hard to discuss. Patients want the hope a new treatment offers, but often the financial risk doesn't outweigh the marginal benefit of the more expensive option. For insured patients, even routine cancer drug costs can mount quickly from coinsurance and copays. If a cancer medication costs $10,000 a month—a common expense, according to the NCI—the coinsurance cost could be $2,000 a month, which is out of reach for many people. Families often help, putting them at financial risk also.

People who are struggling with drug costs may be eligible for discounts or assistance from the pharmaceutical company. Care teams should be aware of discount programs, proactively mention them to patients whether or not financial concerns have been expressed and be willing to help with the paperwork involved. Social workers and financial counselors can be helpful and should be brought in if the person or a family member indicates they have financial concerns.

The cost of cancer drugs can lead to some absurd situations. Jan had excellent health insurance. "The best you can get," her financial counselor said. When she needed an immune booster to keep her on her chemotherapy schedule, she ended up with extra doses she didn't use—and couldn't give back. While in the waiting room for her next cycle, she met a woman who said she was going to have to skip a cycle because her white cells were too low, and her insurance wouldn't cover the immune booster Jan had extra of. There was no formal way to transfer the medication between the women. Instead, Jan and the woman arranged to meet in a nearby parking lot so Jan could hand off the drug, which the woman was most grateful for. "I felt like I was doing an illegal drug deal," Jan said. She was right—what they did actually was illegal. It represents the kind of workarounds our health system forces us into in order to do the right thing.

Financial toxicity may lead some to skip supportive services, such as physical therapy or nutrition counseling, without first talking with their team. Cost concerns include not only copays and fees but also transportation, childcare, and other related expenses. All of these may keep some patients from using supportive and integrative treatments. Helping your patients to find free or low-cost integrative treatments, such as from a community acupuncture clinic or massage school, may be helpful. Some modalities, such as yoga, are taught in low-cost or free settings, such as community centers and YMCAs.

Let people know that financial counselors or navigators are available and can be helpful in planning to meet the cost of cancer care. Also let them know social workers can help them locate free or low-cost care resources and practical support in their community. Social workers can help them connect with community and advocacy organizations that offer free or low-cost help for people with cancer.

MASSAGE AND MANIPULATIVE THERAPIES

Massage therapy is a healing practice that is thousands of years old. It is the manual administration of pressure to the body's soft tissue including muscles, tendons, ligaments, and connective tissue. Massage therapy is typically performed to loosen and relax tissue but can also be performed to treat serious health issues, like chronic pain and lymphedema. The 2022 SIO-ASCO pain guideline recommends massage for pain during palliative or hospice care, general cancer pain or musculoskeletal pain, and chronic pain from breast cancer treatment.

Massage therapy stimulates the body's relaxation and mechanical responses. The relaxation response happens when changes in the parasympathetic nervous system occur. Breathing and heart rate slow, muscles begin to relax, and blood pressure decreases; serotonin is released, increasing positive mood and thoughts. Mechanical response happens because massage increases blood and lymph circulation and relaxes tissues. Improved circulation can decrease swelling and inflammation in soft tissue. As muscle tissues relax, contractions and spasms are decreased. An increase in circulation and relaxation of muscle tissue both help to decrease pain and anxiety.

Within the cancer population, massage has been shown to be effective for breast cancer symptoms including negative emotions and fatigue, cancer pain levels, anxiety and fatigue, and sleep during treatment and for cancer survivors.[10] It can also help with lymphedema for some patients.[11]

Manipulation

Manipulating ("adjusting" is the term many chiropractors use) the spine or other bones and muscles is typically used to help joints to function better by inducing mobility, realigning joints and surrounding soft tissues, and reducing pain sensations and inflammation. The goal is often to correct how the spine bones, tendons and surrounding muscle function, relieve pain, and improve the overall well-being of the body.

Manipulation is part of the treatment offered by many providers, including chiropractors but also osteopathic physicians (fully licensed medical doctors who use manual medicine as part of treatment), naturopathic physicians, physical therapists, and some medical doctors.[12]

In February 2017, the American College of Physicians released new guidelines for the treatment of acute, subacute, and chronic back pain, recommending that patients use nonpharmacologic therapies (including massage, acupuncture and/or spinal manipulation) before trying medication or more invasive procedures.[13] Very little research, however, has occurred on manipulation in the cancer setting. Questions, while theoretical, have not been answered about spreading cancer if skin cancer lesions exist. Currently, the best approach is to be sure that the massage therapist or chiropractor you use is trained and certified by a group like the Society for Oncology Massage (www.s4om.org).

MIND-BODY MEDICINE

Mind-body therapies can be useful during and after cancer treatment and are safe for most people in most situations. Some treatments or activities, such as hypnosis and biofeedback, involve a trained and certified health care professional. Other techniques, such as mindfulness-based stress reduction training, meditation, guided imagery, or progressive muscle relaxation can be taught by an instructor or can be self-taught through apps, online videos, and other resources.

Mind-body medicine can be helpful for both physical and mental challenges related to cancer and its treatment. Mind-body treatments such as guided imagery have been shown to lower the intensity of cancer pain and to help in other ways.[14] Mindfulness training can be helpful with the balance problems associated with peripheral neuropathy.

Taking a try-and-see approach can be helpful. Different approaches can provide the same benefits, but not all are a match for the patient's interests, style, and culture. If it's not a match, try other options. Like physical exercise, the mental exercise of mind-body practices comes in many varieties.

Cognitive Behavioral Therapy

Cognitive behavioral therapy (CBT) is a specific approach to therapy often used for mental and emotional problems, for healing trauma and for treatment of insomnia (even in cancer). It emphasizes how the way we think about something (or perceive it) affects how we feel and act. This approach requires a motivation to change and a willingness to practice new skills (behaviors) and thought patterns (cognition). Patients may learn stress management and relaxation techniques, coping skills, assertiveness, and ways to break unwanted behavior patterns, such as smoking. It is often combined with mindfulness and similar relaxation response techniques.

CBT has been found effective in helping with a number of problems faced by those with and without cancer including depression, anxiety, panic disorder, PTSD, eating disorders, obsessive-compulsive disorder, smoking, and low-back pain.[15]

For people with sleep-related problems, CBT-I (for insomnia) can be very helpful. The data is robust.[16] People can also download CBT-i Coach, a free app for self-teaching CBT-I techniques, courtesy of the US Department of Veterans Affairs.

PSYCHO-ONCOLOGY AND COUNSELING

The field of psycho-oncology acknowledges that the experience of cancer affects the mind and emotions of a person and their whole family. It can address a variety of concerns with a special focus on pain, sexual health, fear and anxiety, and fatigue.[17] Screening for distress can help target which patients are most in need of this kind of support. Referral to a psycho-oncologist or counselor can help your team better address a person's psychosocial needs. Such counseling is becoming a routine part of supportive services at cancer centers. Virtual access is widening these services to smaller clinics and rural areas.

CHAPLAIN SERVICES

As mentioned in several earlier chapters, chaplains can be helpful in addressing patients' spiritual needs. They are essential members of the palliative care team in whole person care.[18] The oncology team can initiate the conversation and offer chaplain services. If someone on your team performs a Faith, Importance and Influence, Community and Address (FICA) or spiritual assessment, you'll know if a patient desires spiritual care, which could come from a chaplain or another source. Opening the door to a conversation about faith or belief in a higher power, or its absence, can allow your team to best support patients as whole people. Spiritual discussions often occur during the HOPE Note process when the team discusses a patient's answer to "what matters" on the Personal Health Inventory (PHI).

Your hospital or cancer center may have a chaplain who can support both you and your patients.

They can[19]:

- Read spiritual material and pray with the person with cancer
- Talk with them about concerns and about making health care decisions

- Help patients' family members with spiritual needs
- Support you and other members of the health care team and providers at the hospital or clinic
- Help the person with cancer, their family, and the health care team communicate
- Create a safe space to deal with loss and grief

Energy Medicine

Bioenergy medicine, sometimes called biofield therapies, includes several different therapeutic interventions where a therapist helps to harness or manipulate a patient's "subtle energy" in order to help restore the body's balance and improve the body's ability to heal. These approaches have been described and used for thousands of years by systems such as traditional Chinese medicine and traditional Indian medicine, and by faith healers through approaches such as "laying on of hands." The most frequently used modern bioenergetic interventions are therapeutic touch/healing touch, Reiki, qigong, and the laying on of hands. Reiki is gaining in popularity and use, largely because of how simple it is to learn and apply. It's inexpensive, safe, and has some good data on effectiveness, so many cancer care teams say, "why not" and provide it. It may also work for many of the conditions more established mind-body practices are used for.[20]

Some of these practices are used widely by nurses and others involved in palliative and supportive care and several have developed formal training and certification procedures.

Mindfulness, Meditation, and Relaxation Techniques

Mindfulness, meditation, and relaxation practices typically go together. Mindfulness is also an aspect of movement practices such as yoga or tai chi. The goal is to learn how to induce the relaxation response for twenty minutes, once or twice a day. Guided imagery or journaling may be useful in managing stress and improving mental resilience, gratitude, and social happiness. We discuss these techniques elsewhere in this book. In this section, we discuss other relaxation techniques easily taught to people with cancer.

Breathwork

The most basic mind-body technique is breathing, also called breathwork. With practice, focusing on proper breathing can induce the relaxation response. Breathwork techniques can be taught by an instructor. They're also easily self-taught using apps, online videos, and other resources. A simple breathing technique called four corners or "box" breathing involves breathing in for 4 seconds; holding the breath for 4 seconds; breathing out for 4 seconds; then holding for 4 seconds in a repetitive cycle. This helps slow down the breath, which helps people relax. It takes very little time to teach this technique to a person sitting in your office or an infusion chair. Try it yourself, then teach it to someone on your team or in your clinic and see the response you get. It's a gift to share a relaxation technique. It's healing.

Guided Imagery

Guided imagery is a mind-body practice that uses imagination and sensory memory to induce a state of relaxation and physiological, emotional, and attitudinal responses. The person is encouraged to sit quietly and remember or imagine a place, activity, or scenario they find pleasurable and relaxing—sometimes described as their happy place. Some people with cancer like to use guided imagery to visualize their treatment destroying cancer cells or to distract themselves during a painful procedure. This can reduce stress, promote healing, improve sleep, lessen pain, and more. Guided imagery with progressive muscle relaxation is recommended as part of the 2022 SIO-ASCO pain guideline for those experiencing general pain from cancer treatment.

Hypnosis

Hypnosis is a widely researched method that is underutilized by people with cancer. Hypnosis is recommended in the 2022 SIO-ASCO pain guideline for people who experience or anticipate procedural pain. In hypnotherapy, a trained hypnotherapist offers suggestions to a patient while in a deep state of relaxation. It has also been found effective in treating symptoms of nausea and vomiting, managing pain, and reducing distress from surgical and medical procedures.[21] It's worth finding out if a mental health provider in your setting has training to provide this service.

While usually delivered by a trained psychologist, social worker, nurse, or physician, there are an increasing number of online resources and apps that can be used. One of the more robustly developed apps is Reveri, created by Stanford researcher Dr David Spiegel, based on his over 40 years using hypnosis with cancer and other patients (https://www.reveri.com/).

NUTRITIONAL COUNSELING

In the last chapter we provided resources that anyone on the team can use to assist patients in learning how to better their general nutritional habits for self-care. Some patients can benefit from or need a formal nutritional consultation with an expert. Helping people with cancer fuel their bodies and modify the tumor microenvironment through good nutrition is part of whole person oncology. Patients who are at risk for experiencing significant weight loss or gain, or who have specific eating-related symptoms like nausea, vomiting, mouth sores, gastrointestinal (GI) cancers, and similar issues should be offered consultation with a dietician or nutritionist as soon as possible.

Patients and their family members often ask us what they should be eating. Take that as a cue to either ask a second-order question such as, "What do you know about food and cancer?" and to make a referral to a professional in the field if that isn't you. Historically, when we don't see the questions as their "bid" to discuss nutrition further, we miss this opportunity to support a person's innate knowledge that food is medicine. We should see the questions as a way to further their healing impulse and support them in any way we can. As more information on the relationship between diet, the microbiome, the immune system and treatment response emerges, the need for more detailed diet counseling will likely increase.

A nutritional counseling consult is usually a 1-hour evaluation to assess the patient. It focuses on diet but may also include assessments of the person's sleep patterns, physical activity, and other lifestyle factors. With this information, the nutritionist works with the patient to identify opportunities for improving the diet and preparing for any changes necessary to deal with anticipated treatment issues, such as vomiting or mucositis. The nutritionist can also help with ideas for eating well when the person has little time or energy to shop and cook. Options could include services that deliver prepared meals or meal kits and discussing healthy choices when eating out. This is also an opportunity to address financial toxicity and food insecurity. The person may be eligible for free meal delivery, local free meal programs, food pantry services, and Supplemental Nutrition Assistance Program (SNAP). The nutritionist can refer the person directly or bring in a social worker to help.

When making a referral, verify that the nutritionist is licensed or certified to practice in your state. The primary organization of qualified nutrition professionals is the Academy of Nutrition and Dietetics (www.eatright.org). The website can be searched by zip code to find qualified practitioners in your area. Look for a registered dietitian or registered dietitian nutritionist (RDN). These disciplines typically require a 4-year bachelor's degree, 900 to 1,200 hours in a dietetic internship through an accredited program, passing a dietetics registration exam, and continuing professional education requirements. Some RDNs are certified in a specialized area, including oncology dieticians, nutrition support, and diabetes education. If someone on the care team has a particular interest in food as medicine, encourage them to learn who else in the community and your referral network shares the interest. Helpful referrals and fruitful collaborations may develop. Interested staff members can also create nutrition wall posters, displays, and other material for the waiting room.

PHARMACISTS AND SUPPLEMENTS

In the last chapter we covered the use of supplements in integrative care. Supplements can both support and prevent healing. Knowing which is the case and how to advise patients can be challenging. That's where a knowledgeable pharmacist comes in.[22]

Pharmacists trained in supplement management can do much more than just dispense medications. Having a pharmacist in a patient-oriented role of supervising the patient's drugs and supplements and providing information and education on medication schedules, costs, and access, can prevent adverse interactions and further support healing. When a pharmacist works at the top of their license, they can better contribute to whole person care. If a trained pharmacist with good knowledge of supplements isn't available, look for one of the growing groups of "tele-pharmacists" to provide this service.[23]

PHYSICAL THERAPY AND EXERCISE COUNSELING

Physical therapy and exercise counseling can be very valuable for people with cancer. These modalities help with recovery from surgery, get people through treatment more easily, and are important for survivorship.

Physical Therapy

Physical therapy is underutilized in cancer care.[24] Some patients need additional support and rehabilitation, especially when dealing with a specific cancer-related impairment or immediately following surgery. Almost all patients can benefit from a supervised exercise prescription. Physical and occupational therapy can help with movement, balance, and everyday challenges. People with peripheral neuropathy benefit from physical therapy to help with balance and fine motor function, such as gripping and lifting objects.

Having a physical therapist on the team can assist with setting goals and integrating movement into the patient's treatment plan.

Make referrals to physical therapy as early in treatment as possible for the most benefit in recovery and for helping any problems that may arise during treatment. One study showed that early physical therapy the day following breast surgery reduced pain levels and improved function without added complications.[25]

Exercise

Throughout this book, we've discussed the value of exercise for people with cancer at every stage of their journey. The evidence for exercise is so robust that all cancer centers should include an exercise prescription as part of treatment.[26] Having an exercise consultant on the cancer team or available for referral can be standard of care. The American College of Sports Medicine (ACSM) Guidelines for Exercise and Cancer and their Moving through Cancer initiative (www.acsm.org) contain information on implementation of these services by professionals trained in exercise.

THERAPEUTIC YOGA AND TAI CHI

You may not think of yoga as a medical intervention, but numerous studies attest to the benefits of this centuries-old mind-body practice on a wide range of health-related conditions, particularly stress and anxiety, mental health (mood problems and depression), poor quality of life, and pain management.[27]

This has led to the development of a new form of yoga that goes beyond just self-care—therapeutic yoga. In therapeutic yoga, practitioners receive additional training in anatomy, physiology, psychology, and other medically related topics to provide personalized therapy to help their clients—your patients—manage chronic conditions. Therapeutic yoga is officially described as the "application of yoga postures and practice to the treatment of health conditions to prevent, reduce, or alleviate structural, physiological, emotional, and spiritual pain, suffering, or limitations." Most therapeutic yoga professionals work or affiliate in hospital or clinical settings.[28]

Numerous studies find therapeutic yoga practice can relieve stress; lower breathing rate, heart rate, blood pressure, and cortisol levels; and improve quality of life.[29] The stretching and flexibility that comes with yoga practice provides pain relief for a range of conditions, along with help for sleep disturbances and depression, as shown by many studies.[30] The 2022 SIO-ASCO joint guideline for pain recommends yoga for aromatase inhibitor-related joint pain and after treatment for breast or head and neck cancer.

The International Association of Yoga Therapists (IAYT) sets educational standards for the training of yoga therapists and accredits training facilities. Standards include 90 hours of training in anatomy and physiology, as well as 45 hours devoted to learning about commonly used drugs and surgical procedures they may encounter, common medical terminology, psychology, and mental health. Overall, therapeutic yoga instructors complete a minimum of 800 hours of training over 2 years, most of which must be provided in person, not remotely. This includes a minimum of 205 hours as a practicum.

Yoga has a low rate of side effects, and the risk of serious injury from yoga is quite small. However, certain types of stroke as well as pain from nerve damage are among possible side effects of practicing yoga incorrectly. Patients with chronic pain can be injured from too rapid or strenuous practice without supervision of a practitioner properly trained for these conditions. In addition, patients inclined to yoga and are looking for it to alleviate certain symptoms may become discouraged if they just do an online course or visit a community studio. Dr Jonas, who frequently recommends yoga, often hears from such patients that "I tried yoga and it didn't work," only to find their symptoms markedly helped by a trained therapeutic yoga professional.

Tai Chi and Moving Meditations

Tai chi and qigong are moving meditations that can build balance, coordination, strength, and functional capacity. Both practices combine the use of slow and deliberate movements with meditation and breathing practice. Tai chi is considered a martial art, while qigong is more of a series of exercises for wellness. These practices don't increase heart rates or burn calories; their main impact is on muscle control and balance.

A systematic review and meta-analysis of tai chi for patients suffering from fatigue found that tai chi was not only more effective than conventional therapies for decreasing fatigue (particularly in cancer patients), but was also more effective in addressing depression, vitality, and increasing the amount patients slept.[31]

Another systematic review and meta-analysis including 499 cancer patients found that those who participated in qigong or tai chi classes had increased cancer-specific quality of life, improved immune system functioning, and decreased cortisol (stress hormone) levels.[32]

Tai chi and qigong practitioners aren't regulated on a federal or state level. Currently, many independent organizations lead trainings and provide certifications to individuals who either take their courses or meet their qualifications. Although there are no official training guidelines, make sure that whatever certification the practitioner holds includes both educational and experiential hours.

The cost of attending qigong and tai chi classes varies based on location, provider, and extent of services provided. Classes can range from free or less than $20 per session at a community center to several hundreds of dollars for an individual session with a master practitioner. If the patient has a membership at a YMCA, gym, spa, or community center, it's possible qigong or tai chi classes are offered. Online videos and classes are also available for those looking for a self-paced, free option.

GENTLY BEGIN AGAIN

Teams should not be discouraged from recommending the self-care practices described in the last chapter or referring patients to the professional supportive and integrative care services summarized in this chapter. Medicine, by its very design, sees more of the problems and failures than the successes. But this is a biased view of reality. Studies have shown that even the most refractory of smokers can and will quit if gently and regularly nudged toward proven smoking cessation methods.

The same is true for all behavior change. The team needs to keep bringing the need and opportunity forward. Jan said for years she wanted to do yoga for core strengthening and liked tai chi. She just never said it to her oncology team. And they never asked her about it. Then, after the fourth of 6 planned chemo cycles, she stumbled and had a nasty fall. Once recovered she called up a friend to do tai chi. That is not the best way to motivate behavior change. Teams educated in the science of behavior change can nudge people gently toward health, healing, and wellbeing. When this happens in routine care, there is healing.

In the next chapter we will show how many of these principles and practices are already embedded in cancer care guidelines. This can help motivate systems leaders and payers to help them occur more easily and widely.

SUMMARY POINTS

- Professional services for supportive and integrative therapies are increasing in evidence and use. They are key parts of whole person cancer care.

- Self-care may also require support by professionals to be implemented effectively.

- There are a growing number of professional services with evidence including: acupuncture, massage, manipulation, music and art therapy, exercise, physical therapy, nutritional and supplement help, psycho-oncology support including mind-body practices, cognitive behavioral therapy (CBT), yoga, tai chi, and others.

- Persistent use of behavioral science works, especially if recommended and championed by the oncology team.

- Pocket guides for many of these are available on the book website.

CHAPTER FOURTEEN

GUIDELINES AND EDUCATION FOR WHOLE PERSON CARE

Professional societies and patient advocacy groups increasingly recommend that various aspects of whole person care become routine for people with cancer. Clinical guidelines often align with the principles of whole person care and its components. However, they tend to be scattered both in how they are developed and who they target for implementation. In this chapter we'll discuss several professional organizations' guidelines that have relevance for the delivery of whole person cancer care. Since these guidelines inevitably recommend or have implications for education of cancer care teams, we also discuss educational opportunities and resources for learning more.

WHAT ARE GUIDELINES?

Guidelines are professional summaries of current medical knowledge and recommendations for applying it. They're published by professional membership societies (such as ASCO or NCCN), national organizations (such as the National Academy of Medicine), private organizations (such as the Cochrane Collaboration), or government agencies (such as NCI or AHRQ). Today, the expert panels that craft the guidelines usually also include input from at least one patient advocate or patient representative.

The figure shows how guidelines are positioned in relationship to delivery of the whole person care as discussed in this book. There are guidelines for supportive care, palliative care, integrative care, patient-centered care, survivorship, and other topics. There are also additional topics important for cancer care not covered by guidelines. In other words, guidelines provide just that—guidance.

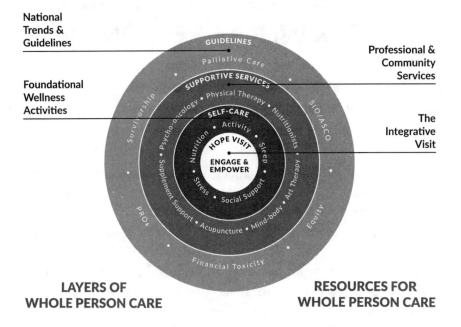

Figure 14.1 The Place of Guidelines in Whole Person Care

This figure illustrates how guidelines for whole person care are increasingly positioned to reinforce the need for core whole person care services. These parallel chapter descriptions found in Part Three of this book starting from the visit in the center (Chapter 11), to self-care (Chapter 12) and professional services (Chapter 13), to education and guidelines (Chapter 14).

Guidelines are usually thoroughly evidence-based and very conservative in their recommendations. They tend to be narrow in the type of evidence reviewed for inclusion (mostly randomized controlled trials) and the standard conclusion in most of them is, "More research is needed." This is true—more research is needed. The narrow focus on the type of evidence used for guidelines keeps people safe when it comes to recommendations around treatment of the cancer. When it comes to recommendations around healing for the whole person, guidelines can be unsatisfying. Such is science and the way we evaluate it.

Unless we tell people with cancer directly about clinical practice guidelines (CPGs), they learn about them randomly—maybe through an internet search or, most often, not at all. Sharing with people that a large portion of their initial care is based on practice guidelines such as those from the NCCN or ASCO pulls back the curtain on how evidence in cancer care drives care offerings. If people with cancer show interest when the topic is broached, such information sharing invites further partnership in care.

In 2016, the advocacy group Cancer Support Community surveyed 1,218 people with cancer to learn about their individual experiences accessing care. Approximately 900 people answered questions related to CPGs. More than half (54%) reported not knowing the meaning of the term "clinical practice guidelines." Well more than half (63%) had "little to no awareness" of whether their own treatment was based on the guidelines.[1] Beyond telling people that guidelines inform much of standard oncology care, we can share the patient-facing materials these partner organizations create as a means of strengthening advocacy through transparency and education.

None of us are all-knowing savants. Rather, we are educated professionals guided by the consensus of expert colleagues. They consider clinical trial data in the context of real-world experience to provide the best guidance they can for the larger practice community. The fact that cancer care is based on consensus guidelines can be very reassuring for patients—they value the authoritative information. For example, NCCN's website states: "The NCCN Guidelines for Patients were downloaded more than 2 million times in 2021." Also in 2021, the ACS's Facts & Figures report estimated 1.9 million new cancer cases in the US. Together, these numbers suggest that people, most likely patients, caregivers, and advocates are looking at patient-facing materials in a robust way following diagnosis. This is excellent.

In cases when our teams exhaust multiple lines of guideline-based therapies, we find ourselves off the beaten path when it comes to the next steps in a person's care. Before discussing with the patient what may be possible now, it can be helpful to trace with them the origins of the standard care they have received so far. At any point in the care trajectory, it can be beneficial for patient, family, and treating clinician to review the CPGs together to share a better understanding of the evidence and recommendations for the treatment.

The NCCN guidelines are also very useful for teaching people about their cancer. They provide some sense of the algorithmic structure of a treatment plan and help patients make sense of it instead of feeling disoriented and overwhelmed—not knowing where they are in the journey.

Dr McManamon often prints out the NCCN surveillance page from the relevant cancer guideline for people who have completed most of their active therapy. It's a good visual reminder of the schedule they've discussed for tests and scans once active treatment is over. NCCN offers numerous patient resources, including patient-facing versions of guidelines for most common cancers, webinars, links to advocacy and support groups, and information about clinical trials.

Guidelines for Whole Person Care

Rarely do mainstream societies such as NCCN and ASCO cover integrative modalities to be used within conventional care, outside of a passing reference or non-ranked listing within an algorithm. This has left oncology care teams mostly in the dark about the safety and efficacy of integrative treatment modalities, including most of the topics we don't learn much (or anything) about in our training: acupuncture/pressure, preventive nutrition, supplements, exercise oncology, mind-body practices, massage, energy medicine and so on—many of the things patients are using or asking about.

GUIDELINES AS EDUCATIONAL TOOLS FOR TEAMS

We're very accustomed to using guidelines from ASCO, NCCN, European Society of Medical Oncology (ESMO), or the United Kingdom's National Institute for Health and Care Excellence (NICE), among others, in conventional cancer care. We're less familiar with guidelines for integrative oncology or whole person care. As we'll discuss, these guidelines do exist and can be a quick and easy way to review data points with patients who ask about integrative and other whole person care modalities. In addition, other guidelines for important topics for whole person care such as supportive care, palliative care, immuno-oncology, the medical home, distress management, and financial toxicity are often scattered across many team audiences and so do not become familiar to the whole team. In this chapter we have tried to bring many of these together to make it easier to use guidelines for implementation of whole person care.

WHAT PATIENTS WANT FROM INTEGRATIVE CARE

An online survey was conducted by IQVIA on behalf of the Samueli Foundation from August 12, 2022 to September 1, 2022, to assess US cancer patient and oncologists' awareness, usage, and attitudes toward whole person cancer care. The survey asked specifically about modalities of care such as nutrition or exercise consultation, psycho-oncology or group support services, yoga, massage, acupuncture, meditation, mindfulness, and spiritual services, among others. IQVIA is a leading global provider of advanced analytics, technology solutions and clinical research services to the life sciences industry dedicated to delivering actionable insights. This survey, consisting of 152 oncologists and 1,004 cancer patients anywhere from 1 to 24 months out from diagnosis, queried respondents on barriers to increased adoption of complementary therapies such as those listed above.

Oncologists (30% academic and 70% community-based) reported divergent perceptions compared to patients when it came to patients' interest in such modalities. For example, 36% of the oncologists surveyed chose "patients are not interested," when in fact there is a known high level of use (and thus interest) of such modalities by people with cancer. Up to 80% of people with cancer are estimated to use complementary and alternative medicine.[2] From the patient perspective, the survey responses were tied at 26% each for the 2 most frequently identified barriers to use of complementary therapies: a lack of knowledge about the therapies and their hospital didn't offer them.[3,4] Fewer than 1 in 5 patients reported *not* being interested in complementary therapies, but that was the primary patient-based barrier noted by one-third of oncologists surveyed. Lack of knowledge about the modalities on the part of both patients and providers, and the disconnect between what providers think patients want and what they actually do want, hampers adoption of whole person cancer care.

The data was telling in the enthusiasm of younger oncologists (age 40 or younger) for integrative care. These younger oncologists identified as being more likely to discuss integrative treatments and to suggest a complementary therapy to their patients, as well as being aware of patients using at least one complementary therapy. In the survey data, nonusers scored higher on items that aligned with a lack of knowledge/awareness as to the modalities and their potential benefits, leading to the conclusion that nonusers especially would benefit from education about the potential positives of integrative oncology. Both nonusers and users of complementary modalities cited the same barriers to use, such as financial concerns and lack of access to complementary therapies at the facility where they received care.

In the IQVIA survey, 78% of patients were Caucasian/white and 10% were African American/black. The experience of black cancer survivors mirrors the survey data. In a cross-sectional survey study assessing the awareness and use of complementary and alternative medicine (CAM) among minority cancer patients (98% black) who were uninsured, the majority (70%) wanted their primary oncologist to provide information about CAM options and discuss their safety and potential benefit for managing their cancer symptoms.[5]

Addressing our shared knowledge gap will benefit everyone. How to do this is worthy of your team's discussion.

Closing the Training Gap

Integrative oncology education is an emerging competency, as shown by innovative ideas such as the University of Michigan's Integrative Oncology Scholars (IOS) Program, funded by the NCI.[6] As an example of "emerging," Dr McManamon, despite a long-standing interest and work within whole person cancer care, was only trained within the pilot IOS Program in 2021-2022. At the end of its initial funding cycle, the IOS program trained 100 US-based scholars. Other programs, in small but rising numbers, are starting to fill the training gap.

The Andrew Weil Center for Integrative Medicine's Fellowship in Integrative Medicine is a mostly online 2-year curriculum open to physicians, advanced practice nurses, physician assistants, clinical pharmacists, and dentists. Up to 180 students have enrolled annually since 2010. Although not oncology-specific, the fellowship led former Integrative Oncology Leadership Collaborative (IOLC) member Donald Abrams, MD, previously chief of the Hematology-Oncology Division at Zuckerberg San Francisco General from 2003 to 2017, to co-edit the textbook *Integrative Oncology*[7] with Andrew Weil, MD and become a leader in the field. Subsequently, the University of Arizona developed an inexpensive Introduction to Integrative Oncology continuing education program for physicians and others in cancer care. This course is a reliable source for more education on integrative oncology and is "designed to provide practitioners with an overview of integrative modalities and treatments that are beneficial for cancer care for patients in active treatment and survivorship, as well as prevention strategies."

Training programs are always welcomed by those looking for more expertise in integrative oncology. They create change in the larger community of practice and begin to close the gap. Yet providing whole person cancer care requires no special credential or training. It's a skill set anchored in the values that brought many, if not most, to work in cancer care. These values aren't always talked about; but when they are, they present as stories of love and hope. Whole person cancer care provides hope to patients and their loved ones for healing even in cases where a cure is not possible. And it gives tools to build back wholeness when cancer is long gone from the body.

Whole person care requires more than learning about integrative oncology and the integration of complementary and alternative modalities into cancer care. But these other dimensions of whole person care still require better "integration" into cancer care to be routine and available for all teams and patients. Adding complementary modalities alone does not lead to whole person care. As Dr Jonas says "integrated" before "integrative." It is this type of "integrated" team training that is needed most now.

WHOLE PERSON CANCER CARE TEAM LEARNING

Whole person care, more so than integrative oncology, requires a period of self-education and a coming together of like-minded individuals on your team to align actions with desired outcomes. To be clear, most care team members don't feel educated on the topics discussed in this book. Continuing to address the knowledge gap in whole person care delivery remains a next-level activity for Healing Works Foundation and other organizations.

Education is only one way to close the gap. During the IOLC sessions we found, not unexpectedly, that the desire to provide whole person cancer care is strong among teams and that application of implementation science lags behind. As lifelong learners, most people in cancer care take in information quickly and can creatively consider how new knowledge can fit into the existing workflow. Implementation then becomes the sticking point. To get to implementation, however, people who work in cancer care need a baseline level of comfort with the underpinnings of whole person care. Guidelines, fellowships, and other trainings can make a difference here. The funding of such trainings (and related additional modalities of care, such as acupuncture to address treatment-related symptoms) remains another issue. Teams can draw upon clinical practice guidelines to ameliorate barriers, both financial and knowledge based. But first, we must know the data upon which these guidelines are built.

THE VA'S HOUSE OF EVIDENCE

In the VA system, acupuncture and medical massage are covered benefits for all patients, based on a robust evidence base for efficacy and low risk of harm. In 2007, more than 10 years before the Whole Health approach to care was rolled out at the VA, the Evidence Synthesis Program (ESP) was founded and laid the groundwork for change. VA's ESP "makes high-quality evidence synthesis available to clinicians, managers, and policymakers as they work to improve the health and health care of veterans." Although not clinical practice guidelines, the many evidence "maps" are available to the public[8] and use similar methods as guidelines (for example, Evidence Map: Acupuncture as Treatment for Adult Health Conditions).[9]

These may be useful as you look to support such modalities for your patients. Because of the evidentiary base for Whole Health, Dr McManamon can refer people with cancer for these covered modalities in addition to conventional care. As the evidence base grows beneath any modality and is incorporated into oncology-specific guidelines outside the VA, the same can happen in cancer care more broadly. We gain more ways to support our patients.

SOCIETY FOR INTEGRATIVE ONCOLOGY AND AMERICAN SOCIETY OF CLINICAL ONCOLOGY: PARTNERSHIP FOR EVIDENTIARY INTEGRATION

A joint effort of the SIO and ASCO is closing the knowledge gap by incorporating the evidence base for whole person care. SIO-ASCO joint guidelines have been developed on topics such as integrative medicine for pain management in oncology and the use of integrative therapies during and after breast cancer treatment.[10] By including nondrug approaches in cancer care, these guidelines provide support for what patients want from their oncologists: recommendations or endorsement for integrative care modalities that are safe and efficacious.

If teams don't have the bandwidth to take on a formal education program for whole person care, clinical practice guidelines can still guide them through the gap. For example, the SIO-ASCO pain management guideline cites acupuncture for aromatase-inhibitor associated arthralgia as a "should be offered" modality, with a 2-point reduction in pain on a 0 to 10 scale. The recommendation is based on data from a sham-control study[11] and led to the additional recommendation that acupuncture "may be offered to patients experiencing general or musculoskeletal pain from cancer." Care teams don't need a personal experience of acupuncture or a deep understanding of traditional Chinese medicine (TCM) to review this recommendation with interested patients. The guidelines let us recommend acupuncture but don't help us find qualified local practitioners or help patients pay for it.

The same issue, as we've discussed elsewhere in this book, applies to other guidelines for complementary care. Typically, there needs to be endorsement and enthusiasm from the team to get patients connected to such services.

Another reason oncology care teams may be hesitant to discuss integrative care modalities or recommend their use is lack of familiarity and comfort with a local network of providers. Building up a list for any community-based resource takes time. If someone on your team is well-suited to this type of research, they could reach out to local, qualified complementary providers to create your referral base.

To bridge the knowledge gap in areas of patient concern commonly encountered in cancer care, additional SIO-ASCO joint guidelines are forthcoming on fatigue, anxiety/depression, and sleep management. Additionally, SIO members were integral in the 2013 publication of the guideline for use of complementary therapy and integrative medicine in lung cancer.[12]

More recently, a 2021 publication out of Canada looked to identify the quantity and assess the quality of complementary and integrative medicine recommendations in clinical practice guidelines for the treatment and/or management of lung cancer.[13]

Lung and breast cancer are 2 of the most encountered solid tumors we face in practice, so it's appropriate that data is accumulating here. The next step may be to move away from diagnosis-specific research to help more people sooner. For example, in an integrative review of the literature from 2016 to 2021 looking at how African American Cancer Survivors (AACS) accept and use mind-body interventions, the authors identified that most clinical trials and qualitative studies exploring complementary and alternative modalities for AACS included only breast cancer survivors.[14] The authors state, "There were fewer articles available concerning male AACS' perceptions or use of CAM but the samples that included both men and women did not report gender-related differences in outcomes."

People of all genders have body-minds. Maybe we move past a parsing out of who will benefit from any one modality and work instead to ask people directly what they may be interested in learning more about. This can be done through a HOPE visit. It may be the fastest way to move past our own biases and assumptions on what may be healing for any one person with cancer.

SUPPORTIVE CARE GUIDELINES

Supportive care plays a large part in whole person care. Your team may be very familiar with guidelines on the provision of supportive care from both ASCO and NCCN. The guidelines continue to expand with new topics such as medical cannabis use in adults with cancer.[15]

Guidelines are constantly being added, expanded, and updated. It may seem like information overload to keep up with them, but they help us improve care for our patients. When working on the business case for a newer or expanded approach to care, use the accepted guidelines to support what you are looking to offer as whole person care. The authority they provide will help move any efforts further, faster among your team and leadership.

To help fill some of the information gaps needed for implementation including summaries of guidelines, safety, and efficacy when available and other information such as training, licensing, precautions, access and payment, the Healing Works Foundation has developed a series of free Pocket Guides to provide a succinct summary of all the main information needed to advance implementation described in detail in Chapter 12. These Pocket Guides are useful for both team and patient education.

Exercise Oncology: An Example

An example of an authoritative guideline that can be used to support your efforts is the extensive work done by the American College of Sports Medicine (ACSM) on exercise for cancer patients and cancer survivors. The 2019 Exercise Guidelines for Cancer Survivors Consensus Statement says, "Enough evidence was available to conclude that specific doses of aerobic, combined aerobic plus resistance training, and/or resistance training could improve common cancer-related health outcomes, including anxiety, depressive symptoms, fatigue, physical functioning, and health-related quality of life."[16] Consensus statements like this give teams strong, evidence-based support for recommending exercise in people with a history of cancer.

One actionable tool the ACSM offers is an "Exercise Is Medicine" (EIM) script, a printable document that helps you and the person with cancer craft a personalized exercise prescription (https://www.exerciseismedicine.org/eim-in-action/moving-through-cancer/).

Within ASCO's supportive care guidelines, the ASCO Guideline on Exercise, Diet, and Weight Management During Cancer Treatment provides related evidence-based guidance based on data from 52 systematic reviews.[17] For people being treated with curative intent, it's appropriate and evidence-based to recommend regular aerobic and resistance exercise. This guideline also touches on prehabilitation (prehab), a growing movement of multidisciplinary care to improve functional capacity and decrease post-operative complications, most often recommended for those who require surgery for cancer. Prehab programs harness disciplines mostly found outside of oncology clinics, such as physical, occupational, and speech therapy and nutritional medicine, among others. Research increasingly supports baseline functional assessment for those with cancer before treatment begins. Changemaking at your institution can come from harnessing such guidelines to drive initiatives such as pre-habilitation to completion.

VALUE-BASED PATIENT-CENTERED CARE: ENHANCING ONCOLOGY MODEL

The CMS Innovation Center's Enhancing Oncology Model (EOM) is a voluntary enrollment program open to practices looking to further whole person cancer care. Through leveraging screening for health-related social needs (HRSNs) and certain data tracking in patients undergoing chemotherapy for seven cancer types (breast, lung, prostate, and small bowel/colorectal cancer, chronic lymphocytic leukemia (CLL), lymphoma, and multiple myeloma), EOM's goal is to improve upon traditional fee-for-service models by funding a pivot to value-based care. The volunteer program is underway with a projected close-out date of June 2028. It is heartening to know that in the US this represents a furthering of learnings from the prior Oncology Care Model (OCM) that took place from July 2016 to June 2022, building on input from participant oncology professionals and patient advocacy groups and aligning with tenets of the reinvigorated "cancer moonshot."

This subsequent EOM states the goal "is for patients to feel better supported in their care; have a clearer understanding of their diagnosis, prognosis and expected outcomes; and be able to adhere to their treatment plan which they develop in partnership with their oncologist."[18] Sounds like whole person care. Services to be rendered and tracked in EOM include patient navigation and care planning, 24/7 access to care, gradual implementation of electronic Patient-Reported Outcomes (ePROs), and activities that promote health equity. Although not a clinical practice guideline, implementation and payment model testing such as EOM will inform what works well and what works less well in the delivery of whole person cancer care.

PHYSICIAN DATA QUERY: WHAT'S IN A NAME?

The large data repository online that is the Physician Data Query, or PDQ (cancer.gov/publications/pdq) is a service of the NCI. As the NCI states, "The PDQ database contains summaries of the latest published information on cancer prevention, detection, genetics, treatment, supportive care, and complementary and alternative medicine." (Disclosure: Dr Jonas is a member of the NCI CAM PDQ.) Most summaries come in 2 versions: a professional level version containing detailed information written in technical language and a patient-oriented version, written in easy-to-understand, nontechnical language. Most versions are also available in Spanish. Boards of experts meet regularly to keep the summaries accurate and up to date. According to the NCI, the boards are editorially independent and "reflect an independent review of the literature . . . not a policy statement of the NCI or NIH."

The PDQs (not to be confused with the Patient Dignity Question) are a great tool for cancer care teams. The PDQ on financial toxicity, for example, reviews interventions aimed at reducing financial distress among cancer patients, supported by citations.[19] It's an excellent tool to spark discussion in a team huddle or education session on finding better ways to address financial toxicity with patients. As the PDQ demonstrates, patients want to have discussions about financial concerns with their teams, but such conversations don't typically occur. A HOPE visit, guided by completion of a Personal Health Inventory (PHI), can bring a concern such as financial toxicity to the forefront and provide space for the conversation to occur. The PDQ is a resource to support patients and teams navigating this conversation.

ELEVATING EXPECTATIONS: THE NATIONAL ACADEMY OF MEDICINE EFFECT

A look back at consensus study reports of the former Institute of Medicine and, more recently, of the National Academy of Medicine (NAM), shows how much the conversation in cancer care has been elevated by this institutional forum for discussion of emerging issues in oncology. Their resultant publications and workshops cover a wide range of topics. For oncology care teams, the best-known publication is the 2006 report that put survivorship concerns on the map, *From Cancer Patient to Cancer Survivor: Lost in Transition.*[20]

When NAM did an update evaluation nearly a decade later in a report titled *Delivering High-Quality Cancer Care: Charting a New Course for a System in Crisis*, little had changed. To quote from that report: "… more than a decade after the Institute of Medicine (IOM) first studied the quality of cancer care, the barriers to achieving excellent care for all cancer patients remain daunting. Care often is not patient-centered, many patients do not receive palliative care to manage their symptoms and side effects from treatment, and decisions about care often are not based on the latest scientific evidence."[21] This is further evidence for the need for whole person cancer care and one of the reasons we wrote this book.

NAM offers a plethora of evidentiary support and elevated expectations for the type of care we can provide. If anyone on your team is looking for subject matter experts to contact, video content to review, or publications to cite when proposing a whole person cancer care initiative where you work, NAM is the starting point.

Another foundational document from NAM is *Achieving Whole Health: A New Approach for Veterans and the Nation*, released in 2023.[22] The document outlines a framework for scaling and spreading a whole health model of care and allows teams to see where progress in whole person cancer care aligns with a much larger strategy burgeoning in US health care.

Separately, as a source of science in the public interest, NAM's website offers a succinct series of articles (also in Spanish) called

"Based on Science—Answers to Everyday Science and Health Questions from the National Academies." The articles cover topics such as what doesn't cure cancer, with titles such as "A healthy diet alone will not cure cancer" and "Dietary supplements will not cure cancer." Each article contains links to reliable sources of additional information for patients and caregivers.

GUIDELINES AND THEIR LIMITATIONS

As valuable as they are, guidelines also have limitations. Because they are put out by authoritative bodies and use complicated evidentiary methods, they often come to be seen as "law" under the guise of "standard of care." Sticking firmly to the guidelines can reduce the flexibility needed for complex, person-centered care. This is especially risky when guidelines are applied as if they were a checklist by inexperienced oncology teams or treatment mills that don't take time to hear the patient. When applied rigidly, guidelines don't acknowledge the reality of uncertainty discussed in Chapter 6, or the nuances of cancer biology as described in Chapter 5, or the importance of patient priorities and empowerment as discussed in Chapter 2. They also don't acknowledge that sometimes a patient's cancer doesn't fit the guidelines (and vice versa) or give much guidance about what to do in those cases. A danger is that sometimes following the guidelines will keep the care team from honoring the preferences of the person with cancer. Our goal in whole person cancer care is always to put the person first and provide the best care we possibly can. In the final chapter of the book, we look at ways to engage the team and implement practice and quality improvement processes that bring in proven methods to make medicine work better.

SUMMARY POINTS

- Guidelines are summaries of evidence, with implications and recommendations for practice made by professional societies and patient organizations to optimize patient care.

- Guidelines have an important role in advancing whole person care. Pocket Guides supplement them with information needed for implementation.

- Examples of guidelines relevant to whole person cancer care include those in supportive care, palliative care, and, increasingly, in integrative care [for example, joint Society of Integrative Oncology (SIO)-American Society of Clinical Oncology (ASCO) Guidelines].

- Guidelines are useful but limited for providing whole person care.

- More educational resources are needed to help teams deliver on current guidelines and other areas for person centered care, including for implementation science.

CHAPTER FIFTEEN

MAKING WHOLE PERSON CARE ROUTINE

We hope that in reading this book you see how you have already been doing aspects of whole person care and are inspired to further advance this holistic approach to healing in your own life, with your team, and for the people in your care. To do so, and to make these concepts and approaches available widely, tools and techniques are needed to help with their implementation. That requires making some changes in health care delivery. For a system ready to make changes, it requires SMART goals and leaders who can communicate the why behind the need for change. Throughout this book, we provide examples and recommendations on ways that health care teams are doing this. We acknowledge change can be quite challenging, especially in a cancer care system historically embedded in a tumor-only focused approach. But can and is being done.

Whole person care will require change at multiple levels—policy, payment, system design, practice tools, and in technology, and health communication. Ultimately, care is delivered at the interface of the care team and patient. This is where the "boots meet the ground" and the endgame of quality health care happens daily. In this chapter, we summarize how changes are made in systems, practices, and individual workflows. In addition, we provide examples of practices making those changes every day using quality improvement, practice improvement and implementation science. We start with one system that initiated whole person care.

IMPLEMENTING CHANGE FOR WELLBEING

In 2012, Dr Jonas and the director of a medium-sized community hospital created a practice improvement initiative to shift the hospital in the direction of whole person care using the framework of an Optimal Healing Environment (OHE).[1] The hospital was in the midst of major renovations and had the ability to link new healing practices with changes in the physical environment. In preparation for this initiative, we surveyed patients and staff on their experiences and behaviors. What was found was instructive for how to shift to a culture of wellbeing in a system. The survey found that patients were highly satisfied with their care and the hospital environment. However, burnout and stress among the staff had increased despite the fact that they now provided care in a beautiful setting. The reason was that the core wellness principles embedded into an OHE hadn't been offered to and implemented with staff for their own self-care, and the demands on patient volume had increased. We forgot to heal the healers and give them sufficient time to be healers too.

Based on the survey results, the first focus of the initiative was to provide core wellbeing opportunities for the leadership and the staff. Leadership further adjusted the physical environment to improve communication and patient flow efficiency, reducing staff time spent finding "work arounds." They made changes such as having breakrooms set up around the hospital and implementation of stress management and mind-body skills training. Faculty development and team meetings allotted time to discuss new ideas for self-care and wellness. Workload and workflow assessments were done to understand where the demand/resource imbalances were and if actual workflow was being captured.

Leadership hired a chief wellness officer. Her time was carefully protected against responding only to crises. She championed staff wellbeing workshops and placed posters communicating the importance of self-care and wellness principles around the hospital and online. A new food vendor improved the quality of the hospital food. Slack time was built into patient scheduling so staff could be well at work. The director of the hospital urged people to take fitness time or stress breaks and had a fitness center built for group classes. Healthy competition arose between teams (for example, number of collective steps taken). The hospital CEO put a sign on her door mid-morning, "Meditating for 20 minutes. In case of an emergency call 911." Leadership meetings and team retreats routinely embedded self-care into their agendas. Mood and morale improved. Improvements in training for coding and documentation of workflow and capture were implemented. Patient navigators were hired and trained to assist with patient coordination and documentation.

Finally, a pilot demonstration clinic implementing an OHE model was established. Through this clinic, staff, resident physicians, and patients could see and experience how to implement whole person care. Inevitably, after rotating through the clinic, other teams wanted to implement some of the practices. Word spread and soon there was a long waiting list of patients who wanted to get their care in the OHE clinic and come to that hospital.

These changes were sustained over 3 CEOs, a remarkable run. Then, the emphasis on wellness and self-care principles waxed and waned as top-level leadership and the economic drivers changed. More than 10 years later, however, the clinic and the infrastructure of self-care still exists, and it has spread to other clinics in the hospital. The overarching lesson of this initiative wasn't that implementing these activities was complex. It was, but how many even more complex practice improvement initiatives are implemented every day in hospitals? The value in economic terms of the shift toward wellness was evident in lower staff turnover, better recruitment ability, and lower costs overall.

This hospital was not unique. Multiple other hospitals have used the OHE framework for their quality improvement practices and report improvement in morale, retention, patient and provider satisfaction and experience.[2] The core lesson is that implementing a wellbeing approach requires sustained leadership to uphold the values that underlie the importance of the drivers of health—for staff and patients.

THE BUSINESS CASE FOR WHOLE PERSON CARE

Still, some hospital administrators are not convinced that whole person care should be a priority. There are so many other demands and forces that displace and distract us from healing. However, there is growing evidence that a whole person approach improves all the key outcomes leaders seek. The business benefits of whole person care are increasingly being studied and documented from multiple settings.[3] One of the largest systems doing this is the VA in which advances in mental health and an initiative called Whole Health (WH) have spread, following its introduction at 18 flagship sites. The WH approach has resulted in improvement in patient[4] and provider experience, retention, improved clinical outcomes, and lowered costs by nearly $5,000 per patient per year. A report from the VA describes these outcomes:[5]

> "Veterans with chronic pain who used Whole Health services had a threefold reduction in opioid use compared to those who did not. Opioid use among WH users decreased 38% compared with only an 11% decrease among those with no WH use. Veterans who used WH services also reported being able to manage stress better and noted the care they received as being more patient centered. These results indicate improvements in Veterans' overall well-being.
>
> The demand for Whole Health services remains high. Over 97% of Veterans responded they were either somewhat interested, very

interested or already using at least one WH service. During interviews for the report, WH leads shared several stories of the impact of WH approaches on Veterans, including reductions in the use of opioids and other pain medications, weight loss, smoking cessation, and improvements in mental health.

Equally noted was the effect WH had on VA employees, many of whom are Veterans themselves. Employees involved with WH at the flagship sites reported lower burnout, lower voluntary turnover, greater motivation, and were more likely to rate their facility as a "best place to work."

Initial findings also suggest that using WH services may reduce pharmacy costs. WH service use among Veterans with mental health conditions (such as PTSD, anxiety and depression) was associated with smaller increases in outpatient pharmacy costs (3.5% annual increase) compared to similar Veterans who did not use WH services (12.5% annual increase). Additionally, WH service use among Veterans with chronic conditions was associated with smaller increases in outpatient pharmacy costs (4.3% annual increase) compared to similar Veterans who did not use WH services (15.8% annual increase)."

The VA started "small" with 18 centers of excellence. Many of these focused first on educating faculty and staff. The principles of whole health, grounded in the core wellness principles described in Chapter 4 and elsewhere, are now spreading to 56 additional VA sites around the country, with plans to become routine at the more than 1,300 VA health care facilities that serve over 9 million enrolled veterans. Whole Health materials are freely available for use (https://www.va.gov/WHOLEHEALTH/index.asp).

Multiple other hospital systems and clinics are implementing these types of initiatives and programs in clinical and community settings. A 2023 National Academy of Medicine (NAM) report documented whole person care models and their value in systems around the world.[6] In addition to the VA Whole Health system the NAM report describes examples of improved experience, provider wellbeing, and health outcomes in systems caring for Native Alaskans, urban city poor, in military settings, and for the elderly. Examples outside the United States were found in New Zealand, Australia, Spain, Germany, Costa Rica, and other places. Whole person care models consistently show better outcomes in patient care experience, provider wellbeing, population health and cost reduction.

APPROACHES TO HEALTH CARE IMPROVEMENT

For those exploring a shift to whole person care at a system, hospital or practice level, there are numerous resources available to help leadership and teams make those changes. One of the most experienced, comprehensive, and time-tested approaches are those developed by the Institute for Healthcare Improvement (IHI), a Boston-based nonprofit that works globally. (https://www.ihi.org/). Their Quality Improvement Essentials Toolkit is highly recommended, for practices large and small.[7] The figure below illustrates an adaptation of their model by Dr Jonas for establishing a Continuous Information and Improvement (CI^2) system that allows for input from all the care teams required for whole person care.

Note that this system builds an improvement infrastructure that is linked to integrated measurement and feedback of the key outcomes needed on the patient experience of care, population health, per patient costs, and clinician and staff wellbeing. The link to these outcomes allows for rapid and real time change as well as continuous determination of value. Also notice the prominent role of "experience experts"—those who are imbedded in the daily operations of the system. The inverted pyramid weights, in which patients and staff have a prominent role at the top, assures that their knowledge and experience—what matters to them—has

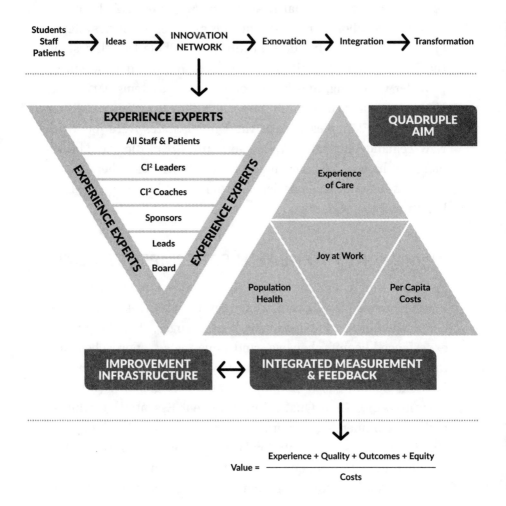

Figure 15.1 Components of a Continuous Innovation and Improvement (CI2) Process for Health Care Improvement

The far left column shows the process used for capturing innovation. Left inverted triangle shows the team members needed for improvement. The right triangle shows the key outcomes to be tracked. The far right column shows the formula for determining the value of the innovations.

a prominent role in any changes implemented. This is the ideal structure and process for implementing whole person care.[8]

Designing an Integrated Practice Unit

One process to test these change principles for whole person care is to design a small test clinic exploring the practice changes described in this book. Such a clinic can engineer a care process in a way that distributes and integrates team members into a more efficient whole. It is an approach suggested by Harvard professor Michael Porter through the creation of integrative practice units or IPUs.[9] This is also similar to an approach for cancer care recommended by Clifton Leaf in his history of the war on cancer, *The Truth in Small Doses*.[10]

IPUs are multidisciplinary teams, ideally co-located and structured to meet the needs of well-defined groups of patients, usually with similar conditions, over the full cycle of care. Oncologists and their teams can create an IPU approach through quality and practice improvement processes. Designing an IPU, then testing and refining it for whole person care, is being done by oncology practice centers throughout the world. Properly designed and team built IPUs free up the time and talent necessary to both implement practice guidelines, as well as provide whole person care. In so doing, they can also optimize use of the best evidence.

Some of the Integrative Oncology Leadership Collaborative (IOLC) members are initiating an IPU approach. Others are redesigning existing clinics that already have elements of whole person care into more efficient practice processes using the HOPE Note Toolkit resources. We have described in other chapters some simple elements that practice teams can use to better provide whole person care such as training in health coaching and patient advocacy; a person-centered case conference; and the Two-Circle Model for Whole Person Care. Several systems have found the Two-Circle Model a helpful framework that advances beyond the OHE vision.

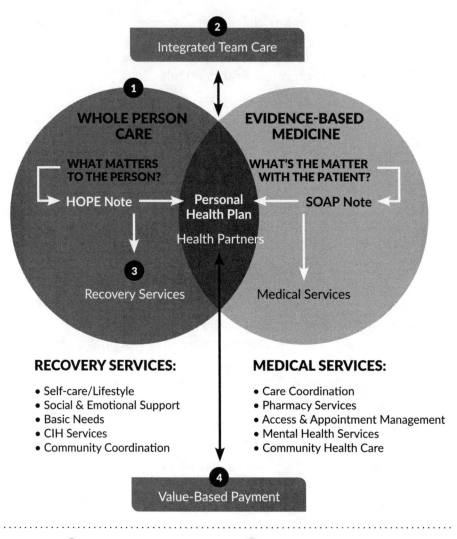

**Figure 15.2 Whole Person Cancer Care Framework:
The Two-Circle Model of Whole Person Care**

The right circle captures the usual tumor-killing processes in cancer treatment with a list of the most common services to the lower right. Left circle captures the person-centered processes needed to make whole person care possible, with the most common services listed to the lower left.

The Two-Circle Model for Whole Person Care

Some cancer centers are reorganizing their approach to formally incorporate patient advocates and whole person care processes into their designs. These redesigns can streamline the use of evidence-based practices and improve the efficiency of care, creating an IPU engine. Figure 15.2 illustrates the Two-Circle Model for Whole Person Care as published in *JAMA Health Forum* in 2022 as an example of such a redesign.[11]

The services in the Two-Circle Model parallel the 2 worlds of a person diagnosed with cancer we illustrated in Chapter 8. On the right-hand side of the model are the activities required for treating the tumor itself. On the left-hand side are the activities needed for person-centered care. The Two-Circle Model integrates both sets of activities through patient advocates and team care, as depicted in the central overlapping areas of the model. This assures that care services listed on the far left are integrated with the cancer treatment plan listed on the far right, and none of them are neglected, when needed.

An example of a system using the Two-Circle Model is the Davidoff Comprehensive Cancer Center, part of Rabin Medical Center in Tel Aviv, Israel. The Davidoff Cancer Center created a Patient Champions Unit[12] to enhance delivery of services on the left-hand side and integrate those services into a personal healing plan for every patient they see. Data on this redesign is being collected on important outcomes for oncologists and their teams, hospital administrators, and patients.

Integrative Oncology Leadership Collaborative

In the second year of the IOLC, 12 cancer centers around the world began to implement or enhance their whole person and integrative cancer care services. These centers were:

- Ann B. Barshinger Cancer Institute, Lancaster General Health (Penn Med–Pennsylvania)
- Davidoff Center, Rabin Medical Center (Clalit Health–Israel)

- DeCesaris Cancer Center, Anne Arundle Medical Center (Luminis Health–Maryland)

- James M. Stockman Cancer Institute (Frederick Health–Maryland)

- Johns Hopkins Medicine (Maryland)

- Karuna Precision Wellness Center (Indiana)

- Life With Cancer, Inova Schar Cancer Institute (Virginia)

- Mayo Clinic Jacksonville (Florida)

- Memorial Sloan Kettering Cancer Center (New York)

- Sentara Integrative Therapy Clinic (Sentara Health–Virginia)

- Sidney Kimmel Cancer Center (Jefferson Health–Pennsylvania)

- University of California at Irvine (California)

- University of Calgary (Canada)

Additional examples of practice redesign by IOLC members varied according to resources and readiness. Here are some brief descriptions:

- The Ann B. Barshinger Cancer Institute, Lancaster General Health (Penn Med) began a quality improvement project in which their survivorship clinic was enhanced with whole person care resources and renamed the "Survivorship and Wellness" clinic.

- University of California, Irvine tapped into the Samueli Integrative Health Institute to embed a naturopathic oncologist into a breast cancer clinic who enhanced their usual treatments with integrative oncology approaches.

- Jefferson University hired an oncologist for their Department of Integrative and Nutritional Medicine who began to offer whole person cancer care support outside of the oncology department. They also began to translate the HOPE Note Toolkit into Spanish for use for their underserved, Spanish speaking populations at the cancer center.

- Dayton VA Medical Center opened a first-of-its kind, tumor-agnostic VA Whole Health Oncology clinic where Dr McManamon uses the Personal Health Inventory (PHI) and HOPE Note Toolkit to offer integrative visits and connect veterans to whole person care services.

- Memorial Sloan Kettering Cancer Center (which has a long-standing integrative oncology center) partnered with Jamaica Hospital Medical Center in Queens, New York, to build a whole person cancer clinic tapped into Jamaica's already robust integrative ambulatory clinics.

- DeCesaris Cancer Center, Anne Arundle Medical Center (Luminis Health) hired additional acupuncturists.

- The James M. Stockman Cancer Institute (Frederick Health) added services to their cancer center to enhance the OHE model they had implemented several years previously.

- Sentara Brock Cancer Center opened the Carrillo Kern Center for Integrative Therapies on site, providing a wide range of services to accompany traditional cancer treatment, from garden therapy to pet therapy to healing touch, yoga, tai chi and massage, among others.

- University of Calgary began a 2-year Integrative Oncology pilot study co-led by a graduate of the NCI-funded Integrative Oncology Scholars (IOS) Program, targeting high-needs patients

- Johns Hopkins breast cancer unit in Baltimore hired an IOS Program graduate (and acupuncturist), to provide integrative health visits.

Some of these settings had tapped into robust quality improvement infrastructures like that described in the CI^2 graphic in Figure 15.1 . Some started or adapted IPUs based on OHE or Two-Circle Model frameworks. Some began to add or train existing staff in new whole person care functions and some simply brought components of the HOPE toolkit into their existing workflow and practice. Whatever changes were made they always involved engaging team members in working together to enhance more person-centered care.

ENGAGING THE TEAM

The key to sustainable changes in health care is to first focus on the staff and faculty. To continuously heal the healers. The midsize hospital becoming an OHE described earlier in this chapter had great ambitions, but soon found no real progress could be made without including hospital staff in the process and supporting changes to help reduce clinical burnout.

When a new institute for integrative care was established at University of California Irvine, wellbeing services were offered first to the employees, staff, and faculty. This accelerated adoption of whole person care changes that had languished for nearly a decade. Now those values and practices are spreading throughout the medical, nursing, public health, and pharmacy schools in the Susan & Henry Samueli College of Health Sciences.

Jamaica Hospital Medical Center (JHMC), a major safety net hospital in Queens, New York, began to implement a whole person care approach[13] just prior to the COVID-19 pandemic, during which they were hit hard. After the pandemic, they brought these approaches to their staff to help them recover. Now the hospital is not only expanding a whole person care model into their ambulatory care centers throughout the city, but they are also working with Memorial Sloan Kettering Cancer Center (MSKCC) to implement the same principles in a new cancer center jointly staffed in Queens by JHMC and MSKCC. To facilitate this process, JHMC is working with OHE expert Lorissa MacAllister, President and Founder of Enviah (enviah.com). Dr MacAllister and her team help hospitals design Optimal Healing Environments and measure their impact. JHMC already works with Planetree International (planetree.org), another company that helps hospitals improve health design. The new cancer center's goal is to be an OHE from its inception.

TEAM SCIENCE PRINCIPLES

As a cancer care team starts talking about how and when to make changes, team science principles can be a welcome guide, particularly because this is not something routinely taught in training.[14]

Team science principles involve how a group becomes a team (shared mental model), building mutual trust, closed-loop communication, and mutual performance monitoring. This last item links back both to inviting people with cancer to give direct feedback as team partners and enabling them to be as empowered as they would like within the planning and provision of whole person cancer care.

Even with these principles in use, we don't always get to a goal in one try. Acknowledging team failure as part of the path to change is important. For example, Dr McManamon is still working to add mind-body services in the clinic, months after an interested ally/research nurse completed the VA's CALM program, a year-long, national mindfulness facilitator training course. The CALM program was designed to equip clinicians with the skills and direct personal experience to teach high-fidelity mindfulness and compassion interventions to veterans. A similar program for the entire medical team is regularly available at the University of Rochester, organized by Dr Ronald Epstein, and is now available as a 7-hour online self-study course (https://mindfulpracticeinmedicine.com/). Team science principles include consideration of what successful teams do. This can involve:

- Coordinating mechanisms: Shared mental models, or how a group becomes a team. As discussed above, patient and caregiver engagement broaden the definition of a team. Make sure to consider who is a project stakeholder and consult them before starting a project. Development of mutual trust—use of clinical pathways and guidelines to inform care is an example of this. Closed-loop communication, including back to a person's primary care provider, when there is one, can occur via a completed survivorship care plan.

- Mutual performance monitoring: Data collection and management, including data-driven QI initiatives that will garner attention and potential funding from the C-suite. Timeliness of care. Feedback from patients, caregivers, and providers.

- Including formal project management in health care: 4Rs (Right Information, Right Care for the Right Person at the Right Time). Doesn't this sound a lot like personalized medicine?

Before you start, identify your project sponsor—a senior leader who provides guidance and makes key decisions. Also identify your project team—anyone who contributes to the execution of the project. Remember to give credit where credit is due, celebrate small wins, and just start. Starting small and course-correcting as needed gets you somewhere. Short Plan-Do-Study-Act (PDSA) cycles are best. The AHRQ has great toolkits and resources to guide you through PDSA improvement processes.[15]

Planning exhaustively typically leads to best-laid plans that don't move forward. Small steps tested, measured, and improved are the best approach.

A good place to begin is the 5-module free CME course on Whole Person Integrative Care (integrativehealthcme.org). While this course was designed for primary care, the tools and practice improvement processes are helpful for any practice environment. A specific 3-hour CME training program for oncology is forthcoming and will be available on the Healing Works Foundation website.

As the saying goes, "a journey of a thousand miles begins with a single step." In this book we have provided the rationale, evidence, implementation tools, and examples so that care teams can bring more and better whole person care to patients with cancer. Those who take that initial step soon find that their actions are more aligned with their values as healers and their systems give more value to patients.

In the process of advancing whole person care, we all become more whole.

SUMMARY POINTS

- To make a whole person care routine requires we change the way we practice.

- Change is always hard, but it happens all the time and continuous improvement is possible.

- Multiple successful tools and resources for quality improvement, such as those provided by the Institute for Healthcare Improvement and Agency for Healthcare Research and Quality (AHRQ) are robust and time tested.

- There is a compelling business case for system leaders to adopt whole person care.

- The Veterans Health Administration (VA), National Academy of Medicine (NAM), and Integrative Oncology Leadership Collaborative (IOLC) have documented many successful whole person improvement initiatives from large systems to individual team approaches.

- This book lays out the rationale, evidence, tools, and examples for delivering more and better whole person care to people with cancer.

- You can begin by taking a single step now.

ACKNOWLEDGMENTS

DR WAYNE JONAS

First, let me thank my wife, Susan Cunningham Jonas, who constantly teaches me not only "what matters" in life, but how that plays out when dealing with cancer. Next, our children are the joys of my life—Chris, Maeba, and EJ—and now the grandchildren, Aiden, Bodhi, and Thea. They are my reasons to seek health and the source of my wellbeing.

Second, while medical school taught me the language of medicine, it is my patients who teach me the meaning of healing. I thank them for the privilege to learn and discover.

Thanks go to my fantastic team at Healing Works Foundation—Doug Cavarocchi, Jennifer Dorr, Lexie Robinson, and Jenny Leyh; to the team at Kevin Anderson & Associates; and to our publisher, Arthur Klebanoff. This book would not exist without them.

I thank Jeff White, Director of the Office of Cancer Complementary and Alternative Medicine at the National Cancer Institute, for his decades of steady leadership and curiosity about healing; Gal Markel, Director of the Davidoff Comprehensive Cancer Center in Tel Aviv, Israel, for his courage to redesign oncology so that whole person care is the central goal; and to Mary Jo Kreitzer, Sabrina Frazier, Nathan Handley, Jennifer Bires, Michael McGinnis, Randy Oyer, and Tina Adler for their detailed reading, input, and feedback on draft versions.

Finally, the space, time, and resources to create this book, and the whole person cancer care initiative, would not be possible without the vision, persistence, and support of Susan and Henry Samueli.

DR ALYSSA MCMANAMON

First, to the Samueli Foundation. Without their generosity of spirit and funding, there would not have been time in this life to contribute to such a project and to have met so many wonderful people, such as my co-author, Wayne Jonas; the high-functioning team at Healing Works Foundation; and the members of the Integrative Oncology Leadership Collaborative, who look to make whole person care a reality.

To my husband, Steve, who makes it all work while holding down the fort, sometimes literally. And to our children, who understand the value of sacrifice for others (or for a book, at least). You are my favorite people and so very loved.

To my larger family and circle of friends, neighbors, patients, and colleagues in healthcare—thank you for allowing me to see myself in you. You all matter.

Finally, to my mentors and co-travelers over 25 years in military medicine. Thank you for teaching me to care for those in harm's way.

A JOINT THANKS FROM BOTH ALYSSA AND WAYNE TO IOLC AND PAEC MEMBERS

The contents of this book drew on two years of discussions and input from members of the Integrative Oncology Leadership Collaborative. Our thanks go to Donald Abrams, Ting Bao, Jennifer Bires, Lara Bonner-Millar, Rita Brereton, Lisa Capparella, Linda Carlson, Tzeela Cohen, Paul Coluzzi, Sandra

Colvard, Terri Crudup, Yehudit Drier, Debbie Fuller, Greg Garber, Nathan Handley, Julia Holbrook, Alison Imboden, Arvin Jenab, Dee Judson, Safiya Karim, Young Lee, Jenny Leyh, Ying Li, Ana Maria Lopez, Gabriel Lopez, Patrick Mansky, Gal Markel, Melanie McCurdy, Kimberly Nelson, Fern Nibauer-Cohen, Randall Oyer, Channing Paller, Chirag Patel, Adam Perlman, Katherine Pisano, Jody Pritt, Jamie Renbarger, Patti Roda, Noga Sela, Jenni Sheng, Wendy Sherman, Jason Starr, Vered Stearns, Cindy Tofthagen, Ora Tzur-Shadai, Barbara Urban, Raymond Wadlow, Shimon Wein, and Jeffrey White.

We thank them for their input and wisdom based on decades of caring for people with cancer. We hope this book will help them advance their teams' goals and work toward whole person cancer care.

We are also grateful to the members of the Patient Advocacy and Empowerment Collaborative led by Jenny Leyh. Members included Louis Lanza Jr, Yolanda Origel, Emily Piercell, and Jasmine Souers. Their voices were essential to guide our work.

NOTES

Chapter 1

1. Prasad V, Mailankody S. Research and development spending to bring a single cancer drug to market and revenues after approval. [published correction appears in *JAMA Intern Med.* 2017 Nov 1;177(11):1703. published correction appears in *JAMA Intern Med.* 2018 Oct 1;178(10):1433.] *JAMA Intern Med.* 2017;177(11):1569-1575. doi:10.1001/jamainternmed.2017.3601.

2. Polley MJ, Jolliffe R, Boxell E, et al. Using a whole person approach to support people with cancer: a longitudinal, mixed-methods service evaluation. *Integr Cancer Ther.* 2016;15(4):435-445. doi:10.1177/1534735416632060.

3. Hanahan D. Hallmarks of cancer: new dimensions. *Cancer Discov.* 2022 Jan 1; 12 (1): 31–46. https://doi.org/10.1158/2159-8290.CD-21-1059.

4. Benjamin DJ, Xu A, Lythgoe MP, Prasad V. Cancer drug approvals that displaced existing standard-of-care therapies, 2016-2021. *JAMA Netw Open.* 2022 Mar 1;5(3):e222265. doi: 10.1001/jamanetworkopen.2022.2265.

5. National Academies of Sciences, Engineering, and Medicine. 2023. *Achieving whole health: A new approach for veterans and the nation.* Washington, DC: The National Academies Press. doi.org/10.17226/26854.

6. Bodenheimer T, Sinsky C. From triple to quadruple aim: Care of the patient requires care of the provider. *Ann Fam Med.* 2014;12(6):573-576. doi:10.1370/afm.1713.

7. Nundy S, Cooper LA, Mate KS. The quintuple aim for health care improvement: A new imperative to advance health equity. *JAMA*. 2022;327(6):521-522. doi:10.1001/jama.2021.25181.

8. National Academy of Medicine. 2023. *Valuing America's health: Aligning financing to award better health and well-being.* Washington, DC: The National Academies Press. doi.org/10.17226/27141.

9. Institute of Medicine. 2013. *Delivering high-quality cancer care: charting a new course for a system in crisis.* Washington, DC: The National Academies Press. doi.org/10.17226/18359.

10. Chong A, Witherspoon E, Honig B, et al. Reflections on the oncology care model and looking ahead to the enhancing oncology model. *JCO Oncol Pract.* 2022;18(10):685-690. doi:10.1200/OP.22.00329.

Chapter 2

1. Remen RN. *In the Service of Life.* Noetic Sciences Review, Spring 1996.

2. Bell SK, Martinez W. Every patient should be enabled to stop the line. *BMJ Qual Saf.* 2019;28(3):172-176. doi:10.1136/bmjqs-2018-008714.

3. Levit L, Balogh E, Nass S. Committee on Improving the Quality of Cancer Care: Addressing the Challenges of an Aging Population; Board on Health Care Services; Institute of Medicine, et al., eds. *Delivering high-quality cancer care: charting a new course for a system in crisis.* Washington, DC: National Academies Press; December 27, 2013.

4. Stacey D, Bennett CL, Barry MJ, et al. Decision aids for people facing health treatment or screening decisions. *Cochrane Database Syst Rev.* 2011 Oct 5;(10):CD001431.

5. Josfeld L, Keinki C, Pammer C, Zomorodbakhsch B, Hübner J. Cancer patients' perspective on shared decision-making and decision aids in oncology. *J Cancer Res Clin Oncol.* 2021 Jun;147(6):1725-1732. doi: 10.1007/s00432-021-03579-6.

6. Trikalinos TA, Wieland LS, Adam GP, et al. Decision aids for cancer screening and treatment [Internet]. Rockville (MD): Agency for Healthcare Research and Quality; 2014 Dec. (Comparative Effectiveness Reviews, No. 145.) https://www.ncbi.nlm.nih.gov/books/NBK269405/.

7. Montori V. *Why we revolt: A patient revolution for careful and kind care.* 2nd ed. Rochester, MN: Mayo Clinic Press; 2020.

8. Kunneman M, Griffioen IPM, Labrie NHM, et al. Making care fit manifesto. *BMJ Evid Based Med.* 2023;28(1):5-6. doi:10.1136/bmjebm-2021-111871.

9. Shickh S, Leventakos K, Lewis MA, Bombard Y, Montori VM. Shared decision making in the care of patients with cancer. *Am Soc Clin Oncol Educational Book* 2023 :43.

10. Ruiz-Rodríguez I, Hombrados-Mendieta I, Melguizo-Garín A, Martos-Méndez MJ. The importance of social support, optimism and resilience on the quality of life of cancer patients. *Front Psychol.* 2022 Mar 9;13:833176. doi: 10.3389/fpsyg.2022.833176.

Chapter 3

1. Barakat S, Boehmer K, Abdelrahim M, et al. Does health coaching grow capacity in cancer survivors? A systematic review. *Popul Health Manag.* 2018 Feb;21(1):63-81. doi: 10.1089/pop.2017.0040.

2. NBME. Health and wellness coaching: How can we support more comprehensive approaches to health care? https://www.reassessthefuture. org/health-and-wellness-coaching-how-can-we-support-more-comprehensive-approaches-to-health-care/. Accessed August 31, 2023.

3. Handley NR, Wen KY, Gomaa S, et al. A pilot feasibility study of digital health coaching for men with prostate cancer. *JCO Oncol Pract.* 2022 Jul;18(7):e1132-e1140. doi: 10.1200/OP.21.00712.

4. Sforzo GA, Kaye MP, Harenberg S, et al. Compendium of health and wellness coaching: 2019 Addendum.*Am J Lifestyle Med.* 2020;14(2):155-168. doi:10.1177/1559827619850489.

5. Khanna A, Dryden EM, Bolton RE, et al. Promoting whole health and well-being at home: Veteran and provider perspectives on the impact of tele-whole health services. *Glob Adv Health Med.* 2022 Nov 25;11:2164957X221142608. doi: 10.1177/2164957X221142608.

6. Smith K, Hays L, Yen L, Wolever RQ. Effects of health and wellness coaching with an adult cancer caregiver. *Perm J.* 2022 Jun 29;26(2):118-125. doi: 10.7812/TPP/21.227.

7. Niazi SK, Spaulding A, Brennan E, et al: Mental health and chemical dependency services at US cancer centers. *J Natl Compr Cancer Netw.* 2021;19:829-838.

8. Richardson MA, Sanders T, Palmer JL, Greisinger A, Singletary SE. Complementary/alternative medicine use in a comprehensive cancer center and the implications for oncology.*J Clin Oncol.* 2000;18(13):2505-2514. doi:10.1200/JCO.2000.18.13.2505.

9. Alyssa Claire McManamon, Marie Thompson. Survivors' stories are the teacher: Narrative mapping and survivorship care plans as educational innovation for pre-clerkship medical students. *J Clin Oncol.* 2017;35(5 suppl):90-90. doi: 10.1200/JCO.2017.35.5_suppl.90.

10. Institute of Medicine and National Research Council. 2006. *From Cancer Patient to Cancer Survivor: Lost in Transition.* Washington, DC: The National Academies Press. doi.org/10.17226/11468.

Chapter 4

1. Sansevere ME, White JD. Quality assessment of online complementary and alternative medicine information resources relevant to cancer. *Integr Cancer Ther.* 2021;20:15347354211066081. doi:10.1177/15347354211066081.

2. Gilligan T, Coyle N, Frankel RM, et al. Patient-clinician communication: American Society of Clinical Oncology Consensus Guideline. *J Clin Oncol.* 2017;35(31):3618-3632. doi:10.1200/JCO.2017.75.2311.

3. Abrams, Donald and Weil, Andrew. *Integrative Oncology* (2nd Edition). Oxford; New York: Oxford University Press; 2014.

4. Smyth JM, Johnson JA, Auer BJ, et al. Online positive affect journaling in the improvement of mental distress and well-being in general medical patients with elevated anxiety symptoms: a preliminary randomized controlled trial. *JMIR Ment Health*. 2018 Dec;5(4):e11290. doi:10.2196/11290.

5. Stanton AL, Danoff-Burg S, Sworowski LA, et al. Randomized, controlled trial of written emotional expression and benefit finding in breast cancer patients. *J Clin Oncol*. 2002;20(20):4160-4168. doi:10.1200/JCO.2002.08.521.

6. Milbury K, Spelman A, Wood C, et al. Randomized controlled trial of expressive writing for patients with renal cell carcinoma. *J Clin Oncol*. 2014;32(7):663-670. doi:10.1200/JCO.2013.50.3532.

7. Deng GE, Frenkel M, Cohen L, et al. Evidence-based clinical practice guidelines for integrative oncology: complementary therapies and botanicals. *J Soc Integr Oncol*. 2009; 7(3):85–120.

8. Ruiz-Rodríguez I, Hombrados-Mendieta I, Melguizo-Garín A, Martos-Méndez MJ. The importance of social support, optimism and resilience on the quality of life of cancer patients. *Front Psychol*. 2022 Mar 9;13:833176. doi: 10.3389/fpsyg.2022.833176.

9. Pinquart M, Duberstein PR. Associations of social networks with cancer mortality: A meta-analysis. *Crit Rev Oncol Hemat*. 2010 Aug;75(2):122-37.

10. Selye H. Stress and the general adaptation syndrome. *Br Med J*. 1950;1(4667):1383-1392. doi:10.1136/bmj.1.4667.1383.

11. Dai S, Mo Y, Wang Y, et al. Chronic stress promotes cancer development. *Front Oncol*. 2020 Aug;10:1492. doi:10.3389/fonc.2020.01492. Doolittle M. Stress and cancer: An overview, Stanford center for integrative health. med.stanford.edu/survivingcancer/cancer-and-stress/stress-and-cancer. Accessed August 31, 2023.

12. Bhasin MK, Dusek JA, Chang BH, et al. Relaxation response induces temporal transcriptome changes in energy metabolism, insulin secretion and inflammatory pathways [published correction appears in PLoS One. 2017 Feb 21;12 (2):e0172873]. *PLoS One*. 2013 May;8(5):e62817. doi: 10.1371/journal.pone.0062817.

13. Dusek JA, Otu HH, Wohlhueter AL, et al. Genomic counter-stress changes induced by the relaxation response [published correction appears in *PLoS One*. 2017 Feb 21;12 (2):e0172845]. *PLoS One*. 2008 Jul 2;3(7):e2576. doi:10.1371/journal.pone.0002576.

14. Mehta R, Sharma K, Potters L, Wernicke AG, Parashar B. Evidence for the role of mindfulness in cancer: Benefits and techniques. *Cureus*. 2019 May 9;11(5):e4629. doi: 10.7759/cureus.4629.

15. National Cancer Institute. Sleep and circadian function. cancercontrol. cancer.gov. Accessed August 31, 2023.

16. Savard J, Ivers H, Villa J, Caplette-Gingras A, Morin CM. Natural course of insomnia comorbid with cancer: An 18-month longitudinal study. *J Clin Oncol.* 2011 Sep 10;29(26):3580-6. doi: 10.1200/JCO.2010.33.2247.

17. Walker WH 2nd, Borniger JC. Molecular mechanisms of cancer-induced sleep disruption. *Int J Mol Sci.* 2019 June 6;20(11):2780. doi:10.3390/ijms20112780C.

18. National Cancer Institute. Sleep problems in people with cancer. cancer. gov/about-cancer/treatment/side-effects/sleep-problems. Accessed August 31, 2023.

19. Savard J, Simard S, Ivers H, Morin CM. Randomized study on the efficacy of cognitive-behavioral therapy for insomnia secondary to breast cancer, part I: Sleep and psychological effects. *J Clin Oncol.* 2005;23(25):6083-6096. doi:10.1200/JCO.2005.09.548.

20. Harsora P, Kessmann J. Nonpharmacologic management of chronic insomnia. *Am Fam Physician.* 2009;79(2):125-130.

21. WCRF/AICR. Food, nutrition, and the prevention of cancer: a global perspective: *World Cancer Research Fund / American Institute for Cancer Research.* 1997.

22. Donaldson MS. Nutrition and cancer: A review of the evidence for an anti-cancer diet. *Nutr J.* 2004 Oct 20;3:19. doi:10.1186/1475-2891-3-19.

23. Fiolet T, Srour B, Sellem L. Consumption of ultra-processed foods and cancer risk: Results from NutriNet-Santé prospective cohort. *BMJ.* 2018 Feb 14;360:k322. doi: 10.1136/bmj.k322.

24. Pati S, Irfan W, Jameel A, Ahmed S, Shahid RK. Obesity and cancer: a current overview of epidemiology, pathogenesis, outcomes, and management. *Cancers* (Basel). 2023 Jan 12;15(2):485. doi: 10.3390/cancers15020485.

25. Milken, Michael. *Faster Cures: Accelerating the Future of Health.* New York, NY: Harper Collins; 2023.

26. Barlow CE, Shuval K, Balasubramanian BA, et al. Association between sitting time and cardiometabolic risk factors after adjustment for cardiorespiratory fitness, cooper center longitudinal study, 2010-2013. *Prev Chronic Dis.* 2016 Dec 29;13:E181. doi: 10.5888/pcd13.160263.

27. Lynch BM. Sedentary behavior and cancer: a systematic review of the literature and proposed biological mechanisms. Cancer *Epidemiol Biomarkers Prev.* 2010 Nov;19(11):2691-709. doi: 10.1158/1055-9965.EPI-10-0815.

28. Patel AV, Friedenreich CM, Moore SC, et al. American College of Sports Medicine Roundtable Report on Physical Activity, Sedentary Behavior, and Cancer Prevention and Control. *Med Sci Sports Exerc.* 2019 Nov;51(11):2391-2402. doi: 10.1249/MSS.0000000000002117.

29. Matthews CE, Moore SC, Arem H, et al. Amount and intensity of leisure-time physical activity and lower cancer risk. *J Clin Oncol.* 2020;38(7):686-697. doi:10.1200/JCO.19.02407.

30. Crudup T, Li L, Lawson E, et al. Awareness, perceptions, and usage of whole person integrative oncology practices: Similarities and differences between breast cancer patients and oncologists. *J Clin Oncol.* 2021;39:15(suppl)e24123-e24123.

31. US Department of Health and Human Services. 2018. *Physical activity guidelines for Americans, 2nd edition.* Washington, DC: US Department of Health and Human Services.

32. Schmitz KH, Campbell AM, Stuiver MM, et al. Exercise is medicine in oncology: Engaging clinicians to help patients move through cancer. *CA Cancer J Clin.* 2019 Nov;69(6):468-484. doi: 10.3322/caac.21579.

33. Sakallaris BR, MacAllister L, Voss M, Smith K, Jonas WB. Optimal healing environments. *Glob Adv Health Med.* 2015;4(3):40-45. doi:10.7453/gahmj.2015.043

34. Sternberg E. *Healing spaces: The science of place and well-being.* New York, NY: Belknap Press; 2010.

35. Timko Olson ER, Olson AA, Driscoll M, Vermeesch AL. Nature-based interventions and exposure among cancer survivors: A scoping review. *Int J Environ Res Public Health.* 2023 Jan 29;20(3):2376. doi:10.3390/ijerph20032376.

36. Tsao TM, Tsai MJ, Hwang JS, et al. Health effects of a forest environment on natural killer cells in humans: an observational pilot study. *Oncotarget.* 2018 Mar 27;9(23):16501-16511. doi:10.18632/oncotarget.24741.

37. Ulrich RS. View through a window may influence recovery from surgery. *Science.* 1984;224(4647):420-421. doi:10.1126/science.6143402.

38. Rosenbaum EH, Rosenbaum I, Perlis CD et al. Creative expression improving the quality of your life with art, music, poetry, and humor. *Stanford Center for Integrative Medicine.* med.stanford.edu/surviving-cancer/coping-with-cancer.html. Accessed August 31, 2023.

39. Bradt J, Dileo C, Myers-Coffman K, Biondo J. Music interventions for improving psychological and physical outcomes in people with cancer. *Cochrane Database Syst Rev.* 2021 Oct 12;10(10):CD006911. doi:10.1002/14651858.CD006911.pub4.

40. Gallagher LM, Lagman R, Rybicki L. Outcomes of music therapy interventions on symptom management in palliative medicine patients. *Am J Hosp Pallia Care.* 2018 February:35(2) 250-257. doi:10.1177/1049909117696723.

41. Schooling CM, Leung GM. Alcohol and health. *Lancet.* 2022;400(10365):1765. Doi:10.1016/S0140-6736(22)02124-9.

42. National Academies of Sciences, Engineering, and Medicine. 2017. *The health effects of cannabis and cannabinoids: The current state of evidence and recommendations for research.* Washington, DC: The National Academies Press. doi: 10.17226/24625.

43. National Toxicology Program. NTP 12th Report on Carcinogens. *Rep Carcinog.* 2011;12:iii-499.

Chapter 5

1. Mukherjee S. *The Emperor of All Maladies: A Biography of Cancer.* New York, NY: Scribner. 2010.

2. Weber-Lassalle N, et al. Germline loss-of-function variants in the BARD1 gene are associated with early-onset familial breast cancer but not ovarian cancer. *Breast Can Res.* 2019 21:55.

3. Hoption Cann SA, van Netten JP, van Netten C. Dr William Coley and tumor regression: A place in history or in the future? *Postgrad Med J.* 2003;79(938):672-680.

4. Esau D. Denis Burkitt: A legacy of global health. *J Med Biogr.* 2019;27(1):4-8. doi:10.1177/0967772016658785.

5. Vázquez-García I, Uhlitz F, Ceglia N, et al. Ovarian cancer mutational processes drive site-specific immune evasion. *Nature.* 2022;612(7941):778-786. doi:10.1038/s41586-022-05496-1.

6. Zhang Y, Zhang Z. The history and advances in cancer immunotherapy: Understanding the characteristics of tumor-infiltrating immune cells and their therapeutic implications. *Cell Mol Immunol.* 2020;17(8):807-821. doi:10.1038/s41423-020-0488-6.

7. Sargaço B, Oliveira PA, Antunes ML, Moreira AC. Effects of the ketogenic diet in the treatment of gliomas: A systematic review. *Nutrients.* 2022 Feb 27;14(5):1007. doi:10.3390/nu14051007.

8. Greten FR, Grivennikov SI. Inflammation and cancer: Triggers, mechanisms, and consequences. *Immunity.* 2019;51(1):27-41. doi:10.1016/j.immuni.2019.06.025.

9. Furman D, Campisi J, Verdin E, et al. Chronic inflammation in the etiology of disease across the life span. *Nat Med.* 2019;25(12):1822-1832. doi:10.1038/s41591-019-0675-0.

10. Hanahan D. Hallmarks of cancer: New dimensions. *Cancer Discov.* 2022;12(1):31-46. doi:10.1158/2159-8290.CD-21-1059.

11. Zhang Z, Zeng P, Gao W, et al. Circadian clock: A regulator of the immunity in cancer. *Cell Commun Signal.* 2021 March 22;19(1):37. doi:10.1186/s12964-021-00721-2.

12. Strøm L, Danielsen JT, Amidi A, et al. Sleep during oncological treatment - a systematic review and meta-analysis of associations with treatment response, time to progression and survival. *Front Neurosci.* 2022 April 19;16:817837. doi:10.3389/fnins.2022.817837.

13. Huang J, Song P, Hang K, et al. Sleep Deprivation disturbs immune surveillance and promotes the progression of hepatocellular carcinoma. *Front Immunol.* 2021 Sep 3;12:727959. doi:10.3389/fimmu.2021.727959.

14. Al Maqbali M, Al Sinani M, Alsayed A, Gleason AM. Prevalence of sleep disturbance in patients with cancer: A systematic review and meta-analysis. *Clin Nurs Res.* 2022;31(6):1107-1123. Doi:10.1177/10547738221092146.

15. Tang F, Tie Y, Tu C, Wei X. Surgical trauma-induced immunosuppression in cancer: Recent advances and the potential therapies. *Clin Transl Med.* 2020;10(1):199-223. doi:10.1002/ctm2.24.

16. Chandler PD, Chen WY, Ajala ON, et al. Effect of vitamin D3 supplements on development of advanced cancer: A secondary analysis of the VITAL randomized clinical trial [published correction appears in *JAMA Netw Open.* 2020 Dec 1;3(12):e2032460]. *JAMA Netw Open.* 2020 Nov 2;3(11):e2025850. doi:10.1001/jamanetworkopen.2020.25850.

17. National Cancer Institute. Stress and cancer fact sheet. https://www.cancer.gov/about-cancer/coping/feelings/stress-fact-sheet. Accessed August 31, 2023.

18. Doolittle MJ. Stress and cancer: An overview. The Rosenbaum Internet Library, Stanford Medicine Surviving Cancer, https://med.stanford.edu/survivingcancer. Accessed August 31, 2023.

19. Bains JS, Sharkey KA. Stress and immunity - the circuit makes the difference. *Nat Immunol.* 2022;23(8):1137-1139. doi:10.1038/s41590-022-01276-1.

20. Hadamitzky M, Lückemann L, Pacheco-López G, Schedlowski M. Pavlovian conditioning of immunological and neuroendocrine functions. *Physiol Rev.* 2020;100(1):357-405. Doi:10.1152/physrev.00033.2018.

21. Jonas, WB, Bierman S. How patients can minimize nocebo effects. In Bernstein MH, Blease C, Locher C, Brown WA. (eds). *Nocebo effects: when words make you sick.* Rochester, MN: Mayo Clinic Press; In Press.

22. Key TJ, Bradbury KE, Perez-Cornago A, et al. Diet, nutrition, and cancer risk: What do we know and what is the way forward? [published correction appears in *BMJ.* 2020 Mar 11;368:m996]. *BMJ.* 2020 Mar 5;368:m511. doi:10.1136/bmj.m511.

23. Liu L, Shah K. The potential of the gut microbiome to reshape the cancer therapy paradigm: A review. *JAMA Oncol.* 2022;8(7):1059-1067. doi:10.1001/jamaoncol.2022.0494.

24. Baruch EN, Youngster I, Ben-Betzalel G, et al. Fecal microbiota transplant promotes response in immunotherapy-refractory melanoma patients. *Science.* 2021;371(6529):602-609. doi:10.1126/science.abb5920.

25. Shah UA, Iyengar NM. Plant-based and ketogenic diets as diverging paths to address cancer: A review. *JAMA Oncol.* 2022;8(8):1201-1208. doi:10.1001/jamaoncol.2022.1769.

26. Terrisse S, Derosa L, Iebba V, et al. Intestinal microbiota influences clinical outcome and side effects of early breast cancer treatment. *Cell Death Differ*. 2021;28(9):2778-2796. doi:10.1038/s41418-021-00784-1.

27. Yonekura S, Terrisse S, Alves Costa Silva C, et al. Cancer induces a stress ileopathy depending on β-adrenergic receptors and promoting dysbiosis that contributes to carcinogenesis. *Cancer Discov*. 2022;12(4):1128-1151. doi:10.1158/2159-8290.CD-21-0999.

28. Calabrese EJ, Dhawan G, Kapoor R, Iavicoli I, Calabrese V. What is hormesis and its relevance to healthy aging and longevity? *Biogerontology*. 2015;16(6):693-707. doi:10.1007/s10522-015-9601-0.

29. Schirrmacher V. Less can be more: The hormesis theory of stress adaptation in the global biosphere and its implications. *Biomedicines*. 2021 Mar 13;9(3):293. doi:10.3390/biomedicines9030293.

30. Furman D, Campisi J, Verdin E, et al. Chronic inflammation in the etiology of disease across the life span. *Nat Med*. 2019;25(12):1822-1832. doi:10.1038/s41591-019-0675-0.

31. Bishayee A, Block K. A broad-spectrum integrative design for cancer prevention and therapy: The challenge ahead. *Semin Cancer Biol*. 2015;35 (Suppl):S1-S4. doi:10.1016/j.semcancer.2015.08.002.

32. McKee DL, Lodhi MS. Natural anticancer products: Classified under the cancer hallmarks and the available evidence of their anticancer activities. *J Cancer Res Updates*. 2021;10:56-81ISSN: 1929-2260/ E-ISSN:1929-2279/21.

33. Drogovoz SM, Starikov VI, Ivantsyk LB, Shchokina KG. Experience and prospects for the use of off-label drugs in oncology. *Exp Oncol*. 2021;43(1):1-5. doi:10.32471/exp-oncology.2312-8852.vol-43-no-1.15583.

34. Anticancer Fund. The untapped potential of unmarketed drugs. www.anticancerfund.org/en/label-use. Accessed August 31, 2023.

35. White CM. Dietary supplements pose real dangers to patients. *Ann Pharmacother*. 2020;54(8):815-819. doi:10.1177/1060028019900504.

36. Memorial Sloan Kettering Cancer Center. About Herbs database. https://www.mskcc.org/cancer-care/diagnosis-treatment/symptom-management/integrative-medicine/herbs. Accessed August 31, 2023.

37. National Cancer Institute. PDQ® Cancer Information Summaries: Integrative, Alternative, and Complementary Therapies. https://www.cancer.gov/publications/pdq/information-summaries/cam. Accessed August 31. 2023.

38. CAM Cancer database. https://cam-cancer.org/en/cam-cancer-database. Accessed August 31. 2023.

39. OncANP KNOW database. https://oncanp.org/know-database. Accessed August 31, 2023.

Chapter 6

1. Leaf C. *The Truth in Small Doses: Why We're Losing the War on Cancer—and How to Win It*. New York, NY: Simon & Schuster; 2014.

2. National Academy of Medicine. 2019. *Caring for the Individual Patient: Understanding Heterogeneous Treatment Effects*. Washington, DC: The National Academies Press.

3. Gunn A, Sarver, M, Kaplan S, Zarfar Y, Greenup RA. Assessing the use of low value oncology care following the release of Choosing Wisely guidelines. *J Clin Oncol*. 2021; 39:15(suppl):e18861-e18861.

4. The National Academies of Sciences, Engineering, and Medicine, Nobel Prize Summit 2023: Truth, Trust and Hope. nationalacademies.org/our-work/nobel-prize-summit-2023-truth-trust-and-hope. Presented May 24-26, 2023.

5. Jonas WB. The evidence house: how to build an inclusive base for complementary medicine. *West J Med*. 2001;175(2):79-80. doi:10.1136/ewjm.175.2.79.

6. Soukup T, Sevdalis N, Green JSA, et al. Making tumor boards more patient-centered: let's start with the name. *JCO Oncol Pract*. 2021Oct;17(10):591-593. doi: 10.1200/OP.20.00588.

7. Terri Crudup, Linna Li, Elizabeth Lawson, et al. The Integrative Oncology Leadership Collaborative Study Group. Awareness, perceptions, and usage of whole person integrative oncology practices: Similarities and differences between breast cancer patients and oncologists. *J Clin Oncol*. 2021;39(15_suppl):e24123-e24123.

8. Samueli Foundation. US Patient & Oncologist Awareness, Usage, & Attitudes Toward Whole Person Integrative Oncology. Final Report: September 30, 2022 (Update Oct 7); Prepared for Samueli Foundation by IQVIA; healingworksfoundation.org/wp-content/uploads/2022/10/Samueli_Integrative-Oncology-Tracking-W1_Final-Report_7-Oct-2022.pdf. Access August 31, 2023

9. Crudup T. Whole-person integrative oncology—A path to improved outcomes and patient empowerment. Open Access Government. January 2023;80-81. doi.org/10.56367/OAG-037-10637.

10. Brandhorst S. Fasting and fasting-mimicking diets for chemotherapy augmentation. *Geroscience*. 2021 Jun;43(3):1201-1216. doi: 10.1007/s11357-020-00317-7

11. Jonas WB, Bierman S. How patients can minimize nocebo effects. In Bernstein MH, Blease C, Locher C, Brown WA. (eds). *The Nocebo Effect: When Words Make You Sick*. Rochester, MN: Mayo Clinic Press; In Press.

12. Colloca L, Barsky AJ. Placebo and nocebo effects. *N Engl J Med*. 2020;382(6):554-561. doi:10.1056/NEJMra1907805.

13. Nestoriuc Y, von Blanckenburg P, Schuricht F, et al. Is it best to expect the worst? Influence of patients' side-effect expectations on endocrine

treatment outcome in a 2-year prospective clinical cohort study. *Ann Oncol.* 2016;27(10):1909-1915. doi:10.1093/annonc/mdw266.

14. Bierman, S. *Healing Beyond Pills & Potions: Core Principles for Helpers & Healers.* California: Gyro Press International; 2020.

15. Mukherjee S. *The Laws of Medicine: Field Notes from an Uncertain Science.* Simon & Schuster/TED; 2015.

Chapter 7

1. Earnest M. When cancer cured pain. *N Engl J Med.* 2023;388(10):870-871. doi:10.1056/NEJMp2215223.

2. Oberoi S, Yang J, Woodgate RL, et al. Association of mindfulness-based interventions with anxiety severity in adults with cancer: A systematic review and meta-analysis. *JAMA Netw Open.* 2020 Aug 3;3(8):e2012598. doi:10.1001/jamanetworkopen.2020.12598.

3. Mannion S, Martin NA, O'Connor J, Wieland J, Jatoi A. In their own words, "Waiting sucks:" A qualitative study of medical testing-related anxiety in patients with cancer. *Am J Hosp Palliat Care.* 2023 May;40(5):468-474. doi: 10.1177/10499091221105502.

4. Holder TRN, Gruen ME, Roberts DL, Somers T, Bozkurt A. A systematic literature review of animal-assisted interventions in oncology (part I): Methods and results. *Integr Cancer Ther.* 2020 Jan-Dec;19:1534735420943278. doi: 10.1177/1534735420943278.

5. Berry LL, Danaher TS, Chapman RA, Awdish RLA. Role of kindness in cancer care. *J Oncol Pract.* 2017;13(11):744-750. doi:10.1200/JOP.2017.026195.

6. Allegra CJ, Hall R, Yothers G. Prevalence of burnout in the US oncology community: Results of a 2003 survey. *J Oncol Pract.* 2005 Nov;1(4):140-7. doi: 10.1200/JOP.2005.1.4.140.

7. Gajra A, Bapat B, Jeune-Smith Y, et al. Frequency and Causes of Burnout in US Community Oncologists in the Era of Electronic Health Records. *JCO Oncol Pract.* 2020;16(4):e357-e365. doi:10.1200/JOP.19.

8. Prevalence of and Factors Associated With Nurse Burnout in the US. *JAMA Netw Open.* 2021;4(2):e2036469. doi:10.1001/jamanetworkopen.2020.36469

9. The Remen Institute for the Study of Health & Illness (RISHI). rishiprograms.org. Accessed August 31, 2023.

10. Epstein R. *Attending: Medicine, mindfulness, and humanity.* New York, NY: Scribner; 2018.

11. Jampolsky GG. *Love is letting go of fear.* Celestial Arts (3rd ed.); 2010.

12. Pinquart M, Duberstein PR. Associations of social networks with cancer mortality: A meta-analysis. *Crit Rev Oncol Hematol.* 2010;75(2):122-137.

13. Katsaros D, Hawthorne J, Patel J, Pothier K, Aungst T, Franzese C. Optimizing social support in oncology with digital platforms. *JMIR Cancer.* 2022;8(2):e36258. doi: 10.2196/36258.

14. Dai S, Mo Y, Wang Y, Xiang B, et al. Chronic stress promotes cancer development. *Front Oncol.* 2020 Aug 19;10:1492. doi: 10.3389/fonc.2020.01492.

15. Jacobson JO, Rotenstein LS, Berry LL. New diagnosis bundle: Improving care delivery for patients with newly diagnosed cancer. *J Oncol Pract.* 2016 May;12(5):404-6. doi: 10.1200/JOP.2016.011163.

16. Barberan Parraga C, Singh R, et al. Colorectal cancer screening disparities among race: A zip code level analysis. *Clin Colorectal Cancer.* 2023;22(2):183-189. doi:10.1016/j.clcc.2023.01.001.

17. Kratzer TB, Jemal A, Miller KD, et al. Cancer statistics for American Indian and Alaska Native individuals, 2022: Including increasing disparities in early onset colorectal cancer. *CA A Cancer J Clin.* 2023;73:120-146. doi.org/10.3322/caac.21757.

18. Ndugga N, Artiga S. Disparities in health and health care: Five key questions and answers. KFF Issue Brief, April 21, 2023. kff.org/racial-equity-and-health-policy/issue-brief/disparities-in-health-and-health-care-5-key-question-and-answers/. Accessed August 31, 2023.

Chapter 8

1. Schear RM, Eckhardt SG, Richardson R, Jones B, Kvale E. Cancer Life reiMagined: The CaLM Model of whole-person cancer care. *Oncol Issues.* 2020;35(4):22-35."

2. Etienne G, Guilhot J, Rea D, et al. Long-term follow-up of the French stop Imatinib (STIM1) study in patients with chronic myeloid leukemia. *J Clin Oncol.* 2017;35(3):298-305. doi:10.1200/JCO.2016.68.2914.

3. Okada M, Imagawa J, Tanaka H, et al. Final 3-year results of the dasatinib discontinuation trial in patients with chronic myeloid leukemia who received dasatinib as a second-line treatment. *Clin Lymphoma Myeloma Leuk.* 2018;18(5):353-360.e1. doi:10.1016/j.clml.2018.03.004.

4. Topal H, Aerts R, Laenen A, et al. Survival after minimally invasive vs open surgery for pancreatic adenocarcinoma. *JAMA Netw Open.* 2022;5(12):e2248147. doi:10.1001/jamanetworkopen.2022.48147

5. Kunkler IH, Williams LJ et al. breast-conserving surgery with or without irradiation in early breast cancer. *N Engl J Med.* 2023;388:585-594. doi: 10.1056/NEJMoa2207586.

6. Coles CE, Haviland JS, Kirby AM, et al. Dose-escalated simultaneous integrated boost radiotherapy in early breast cancer (IMPORT HIGH): A multicentre, phase 3, non-inferiority, open-label, randomised controlled trial. *Lancet.* 2023;401(10394):2124-2137. doi:10.1016/S0140-6736(23)00619-0.

7. Noel L, Phillips F, Tossas-Milligan K, et al. Community-academic partnerships: Approaches to engagement. *Am Soc Clin Oncol Educ Book.* 2019 Jan;39:88-95. doi: 10.1200/EDBK_246229.

8. Aaron Martin as told to Jo Cavallo, "Grieving the Loss of Sexual Intimacy as a Result of Cancer and Its Treatment." *The ASCO Post*, March 10, 2022.

9. Riviere P, Luterstein E, Kumar A, et al. Survival of African American and non-Hispanic white men with prostate cancer in an equal-access health care system. *Cancer*. 2020;126(8):1683-1690. doi:10.1002/cncr.32666.

10. Safdie FM, Dorff T, Quinn D, et al. Fasting and cancer treatment in humans: A case series report. *Aging (Albany NY)*. 2009 Dec 31;1(12):988-1007. doi:10.18632/aging.100114.

11. Cohen S. The nocebo effect of informed consent. *Bioethics*. 2014;28(3):147-154. doi:10.1111/j.1467-8519.2012.01983.

12. Gelfand S. The nocebo effect and informed consent-taking autonomy seriously. *Camb Q Health Ethics*. 2020;29(2):223-235. doi:10.1017/S0963180119001026.

13. Bleicher R. Delay in breast cancer treatment: Is it harmful? 22nd Annual Lynn Sage Breast Cancer Symposium. Presented September 11, 2020.

14. Grossmann NC, Rajwa P, Quhal F, et al. Comparative outcomes of primary versus recurrent high-risk non-muscle-invasive and primary versus secondary muscle-invasive bladder cancer after radical cystectomy: Results from a retrospective multicenter study. *Eur Urol Open Sci*. 2022 Apr 1;39:14-21. doi:10.1016/j.euros.2022.02.011.

15. Poletajew S, Lisiński J, Moskal K, et al. The time from diagnosis of bladder cancer to radical cystectomy in Polish urological centres: Results of CysTiming Poland study. *Cent European J Urol*. 2014;67(4):329-332. doi:10.5173/ceju.2014.04.art2.

16. Weber DD, Aminzadeh-Gohari S, Tulipan J, et al. Ketogenic diet in the treatment of cancer - Where do we stand? *Mol Metab*. 2020 Mar;33:102-121. doi: 10.1016/j.molmet.2019.06.026.

17. Vernieri C, Fucà G, Ligorio F, et al. Fasting-Mimicking Diet Is Safe and Reshapes Metabolism and Antitumor Immunity in Patients with Cancer. *Cancer Discov*. 2022;12(1):90-107. doi:10.1158/2159-8290. CD-21-0030

18. hooks b. *All About Love*. New York, NY: William Morrow and Company; 2018.

Chapter 9

1. Institute of Medicine, National Research Council; M Hewitt, S Greenfield, E Stoval, eds. *From Cancer Patient to Cancer Survivor: Lost in Transition*. Washington, DC: The National Academies Press; 2006.

2. American Cancer Society. *Cancer Treatment & Survivorship Facts & Figures 2022-2024*. Atlanta: American Cancer Society. 2022.

3. Gallicchio L, Devasia TP, Tonorezos E, Mollica MA, Mariotto A. Estimation of the number of individuals living with metastatic cancer in the United States. *JNCI*. 2022 Aug;112(11):1476-1483. doi: 10.1093/jnci/djac158.

4. Neo J, Fettes L, Gao W, Higginson IJ, Maddocks M. Disability in activities of daily living among adults with cancer: a systematic review and meta-analysis. *Cancer Treat Rev.* 2017;61:94-106.

5. Pergolotti M, Deal AM, Lavery J, Reeve BB, Muss HB. The prevalence of potentially modifiable functional deficits and the subsequent use of occupational and physical therapy by older adults with cancer. *J Geriatr Oncol.* 2015;6:194-201.

6. NCCN Clinical Practice Guidelines in Oncology: Survivorship. Version 1. 2023, March 24, 2023.

7. Radhakrishnan A, Chandler McLeod M, Hamilton AS, Ward KC, Katz SJ, Hawley ST, Wallner LP. Preferences for physician roles in follow-up care during survivorship: Do patients, primary care providers, and oncologists agree? *J Gen Intern Med.* 2019 Feb;34(2):184-186. doi: 10.1007/s11606-018-4690-5.

8. Hill RE, Wakefield CE, Cohn RJ, et al. Survivorship care plans in cancer: A meta-analysis and systematic review of care plan outcomes. *Oncologist.* 2020 Feb;25(2):e351-e372. doi: 10.1634/theoncologist.2019-0184.

9. Blanchard CM, Courneya KS, Stein K, American Cancer Society's SCS, II. Cancer survivors' adherence to lifestyle behavior recommendations and associations with health-related quality of life: Results from the American Cancer Society's SCS-II. *J Clin Oncol.* 2008;26:2198–2204.

10. Kwan ML, Weltzien E, Kushi LH, et al. Dietary patterns and breast cancer recurrence and survival among women with early-stage breast cancer. *J Clin Oncol.* 2009 Feb 20;27(6):919-26. doi: 10.1200/JCO.2008.19.4035.

11. Wang F, Cai H, Gu K, et al. Adherence to dietary recommendations among long-term breast cancer survivors and cancer outcome associations. *Cancer Epidemiol Biomarkers Prev.* 2020 Feb;29(2):386-395. doi: 10.1158/1055-9965.EPI-19-0872.

12. Burden S, Jones DJ, Sremanakova J, et al. Dietary interventions for adult cancer survivors. *Cochrane Database Syst Rev.* 2019 Nov 22;2019(11):CD011287. doi: 10.1002/14651858.CD011287.pub2.

13. Van Blarigan EL, Fuchs CS, Niedzwiecki D, et al. The Alliance Trail Clinical Group. Association of survival with adherence to the American Cancer Society Nutrition and Physical Activity Guidelines for Cancer Survivors after colon cancer diagnosis: The CALGB 89803/Alliance Trial. [Erratum in: JAMA Oncol. 2019 Apr 1;5(4):579.] *JAMA Oncol.* 2018 Jun 1;4(6):783-790. doi: 10.1001/jamaoncol.2018.0126.

14. Cannioto RA, Hutson A, Dighe S, et al. Physical activity before, during, and after chemotherapy for high-risk breast cancer: Relationships with survival. *J Natl Cancer Inst.* 2021 Jan 4;113(1):54–63. doi: 10.1093/jnci/djaa046.

15. Campbell KL, Winters-Stone KM, Wiskemann J, et al. Exercise guidelines for cancer survivors: consensus statement from international multidisciplinary roundtable. *Med Sci Sports Exerc.* 2019 Nov;51(11):2375-2390. doi: 10.1249/MSS.0000000000002116.

16. Moris C, Wonders KY. What we know now: Concise review on the safety of exercise on symptoms of lymphedema. *World J Clin Oncol.* 2015;6(4):43-44.

17. Schmitz KH, Campbell AM, Stuiver MM, et al. Exercise is medicine in oncology: Engaging clinicians to help patients move through cancer. *CA Cancer J Clin.* 2019 Nov;69(6):468-484. doi: 10.3322/caac.21579.

18. Heston AH, Schwartz AL, Justice-Gardiner H, Hohman KH. Addressing physical activity needs of survivors by developing a community-based exercise program: LIVESTRONG at the YMCA. *Clin J Oncol Nurs.* 2015;19:213–217. doi: 10.1188/15.CJON.213-217.

19. Gallaway MS, Townsend JS, Shelby D, Puckett MC. Pain among cancer survivors. Prev *Chronic Dis.* 2020;17:190367. doi: 10.5888/pcd17.190367.

20. Jiang C, Wang H, Wang Q, Luo Y, Sidlow R, Han X. Prevalence of chronic pain and high-impact chronic pain in cancer survivors in the United States. *JAMA Oncol.* 2019;5(8):1224-1226. doi:10.1001/jamaoncol.2019.1439.

21. Smith TG, Troeschel AN, Castro KM, et al. Perceptions of patients with breast and colon cancer of the management of cancer-related pain, fatigue, and emotional distress in community oncology. *J Clin Oncol.* 2019;37(19):1666-1676. doi:10.1200/JCO.18.01579.

22. Mao JJ, Ismaila N, Bao T, Barton D, et al. Integrative medicine for pain management in oncology: Society for Integrative Oncology-ASCO Guideline. *J Clin Oncol.* 2022 Dec 1;40(34):3998-4024. doi: 10.1200/JCO.22.01357.

23. National Comprehensive Cancer Network. *Cancer-Related Fatigue. Version 2.2023.*

24. McMillan EM, Newhouse IJ. Exercise is an effective treatment modality for reducing cancer-related fatigue and improving physical capacity in cancer patients and survivors: a meta-analysis. *Appl Physiol Nutr Metab.* 2011;36:892-903.

25. Cramer H, Lauche R, Klose P, et al. Yoga for improving health related quality of life, mental health and cancer-related symptoms in women diagnosed with breast cancer. *Cochrane Database Syst Rev.* 2017;1:CD010802.

26. Wayne PM, Lee MS, Novakowski J, et al. Tai chi and qi gong for cancer-related symptoms and quality of life: A systematic review and meta-analysis. *J Cancer Surviv.* 2018;12:256-267.

27. Kinkead B, Schettler PJ, Larson ER, et al. Massage therapy decreases cancer-related fatigue: Results from a randomized early phase trial. *Cancer.* 2018;124:546-554.

28. Ling WM, Lui LY, So WK, Chan K. Effects of acupuncture and acupressure on cancer-related fatigue: a systematic review. *Oncol Nurs Forum.* 2014;41:581-592.

29. Goedendorp MM, Gielissen MF, Verhagen CA, Bleijenberg G. Psychosocial interventions for reducing fatigue during cancer treatment in adults. *Cochrane Database Syst Rev.* 2009:CD006953.

30. Johns SA, Brown LF, Beck-Coon K, Monahan PO, Tong Y, Kroenke K. Randomized controlled pilot study of mindfulness-based stress reduction for persistently fatigued cancer survivors. *Psychooncology.* 2015 Aug;24(8):885-93. doi: 10.1002/pon.3648.

31. Strollo SE, Fallon EA, Gapstur SM, Smith TG. Cancer-related problems, sleep quality, and sleep disturbance among long-term cancer survivors at 9-years post diagnosis. *Sleep Med.* 2020;65:177-185. doi:10.1016/j.sleep.2019.10.008.

32. Lim CS, Davies AH. Graduated compression stockings. *CMAJ.* 2014;186(10):E391-E398. doi:10.1503/cmaj.131281/.

33. Ezzo J, Manheimer E, McNeely ML, et al. Manual lymphatic drainage for lymphedema following breast cancer treatment. *Cochrane Database Syst Rev.* 2015 May 21;(5):CD003475. doi:10.1002/14651858.CD003475.pub2.

34. Moris C, Wonders KY. What we know now: Concise review on the safety of exercise on symptoms of lymphedema. *World J Clin Oncol.* 2015;6(4):43-44.

35. Janelsins MC, Kesler SR, Ahles TA, Morrow GR. Prevalence, mechanisms, and management of cancer-related cognitive impairment. *Int Rev Psychiatry.* 2014;26(1):102-113. doi:10.3109/09540261.2013.864260.

36. Andersen BL, Lacchetti C, Ashing K, et al. Management of Anxiety and Depression in Adult Survivors of Cancer: ASCO Guideline Update. *J Clin Oncol.* 2023 Jun 20;41(18):3426-3453. doi: 10.1200/JCO.23.00293.

37. Given BA, Sherwood P, Given CW. Support for caregivers of cancer patients: transition after active treatment. *Cancer Epidemiol Biomarkers Prev.* 2011; 20: 2015- 2021.

38. McManamon AC. Survivors' stories are the teacher: Narrative mapping and survivorship care plans as educational innovation for pre-clerkship medical students. *J Clin Oncol.* 2017 Mar 21; 35(5suppl):90-90.

39. Andac-Jones E, Gonzalo M, Kelly G, Weldon S. Impact of integrative therapies on patients with metastatic breast cancer. Poster presentation. San Antonio Breast Cancer Symposium 2022. https://uniteforher.org/sabcs/. Accessed August 31, 2023.

Chapter 10

1. Wachterman MW, Sommers BD. Dying poor in the US—disparities in end-of-life care. *JAMA.* 2021;325(5):423–424. doi:10.1001/jama.2020.26162.

2. Mulville AK, Widick NN, Makani NS. Timely referral to hospice care for oncology patients: A retrospective review. Am J Hosp Palliat Care. 2019 Jun;36(6):466-471. doi: 10.1177/1049909118820494.

3. Goodman DC, Morden NE, Chang CH, et al. Trends in Cancer Care Near the End of Life: A Dartmouth Atlas of Health Care Brief. Lebanon (NH): The Dartmouth Institute for Health Policy and Clinical Practice; 2013 Sep 4. Trends in Cancer Care Near the End of Life. Available from: https://www.ncbi.nlm.nih.gov/books/NBK586638/. Accessed August 31. 2023.

4. Sullivan DR, Chan B, Lapidus JA, et al. Association of early palliative care use with survival and place of death among patients with advanced lung cancer receiving care in the Veterans Health Administration. *JAMA Oncol.* 2019;5(12):1702–1709. doi:10.1001/jamaoncol.2019.3105.

5. Temel JS, Greer JA, Muzikansky A, et al. Early palliative care for patients with metastatic non-small-cell lung cancer. *N Engl J Med.* 2010;363(8):733-742. doi:10.1056/NEJMoa1000678.

6. Antunes ML, Reis-Pina P. The physician and end-of-life spiritual care: The PALliatiVE Approach. *Am J Hospice Palliat Med.* 2022;39(10):1215-1226. doi:10.1177/10499091211068819

7. Borneman T, Ferrell B, Puchalski CM. Evaluation of the FICA tool for spiritual assessment. *J Pain Symptom Manage.* 2010;40(2):163-173. doi:10.1016/j.jpainsymman.2009.12.019.

8. Jonas WB, Jonas M. 2019. *Faith-health collaboration to improve community and population health. NAM Perspectives.* Commentary, National Academy of Medicine, Washington, DC. doi.org/10.31478/201908a.

9. Ameli R, Sinaii N, Luna MJ, Cheringal J, Gril B, Berger A. The National Institutes of Health measure of Healing Experience of All Life Stressors (NIH-HEALS): Factor analysis and validation. *PLoS One.* 2018 Dec 12;13(12):e0207820. doi:10.1371/journal.pone.0207820.

10. Dingley C, Ruckdeschel A, Kotula K, Lekhak N. Implementation and outcomes of complementary therapies in hospice care: an integrative review. *Palliat Care Soc Pract.* 2021 Oct 26;15:26323524211051753. doi:10.1177/26323524211051753.

11. Tabatabaee A, Tafreshi MZ, Rassouli M, et al. Effect of therapeutic touch in patients with cancer: A literature review. *Med Arch.* 2016;70(2):142-147. doi:10.5455/medarh.2016.70.142-147.

12. Gyawali B, Eisenhauer E, Tregear M, Booth CM. Progression-free survival: It is time for a new name. Lancet Oncol. 2022 Mar;23(3):328-330. doi: 10.1016/S1470-2045(22)00015-8.

13. Cohen MG, Althouse AD, Arnold RM, et al. Hope and advance care planning in advanced cancer: Is there a relationship? *Cancer.* 2022 Mar 15;128(6):1339-1345. doi: 10.1002/cncr.34034.

14. Robinson CA. "Our best hope is a cure." Hope in the context of advance care planning. *Palliat Support Care.* 2012 Jun;10(2):75-82. doi: 10.1017/S147895151100068X.

15. Serey K, Cambriel A, Pollina-Bachellerie A, Lotz JP, Philippart F. Advance directives in oncology and haematology: A long way to go-a

narrative review. *J Clin Med.* 2022 Feb 23;11(5):1195. doi: 10.3390/jcm11051195.

16. Maciejewski PK, Phelps AC, Kacel EL, et al. Religious coping and behavioral disengagement: opposing influences on advance care planning and receipt of intensive care near death. *Psychooncology.* 2012; 21(7):714-723. doi:10.1002/pon.1967.

17. Dignity in Care. Patient dignity questionnaire, PDQ. www.dignityincare.ca/en/the-patient-dignity-question-html. Accessed August 31, 2023.

18. American Childhood Cancer Association. US childhood cancer statistics. www.acco.org/us-childhood-cancer-statistics. Accessed August 31, 2023.

19. Linebarger JS, Johnson V, Boss RD, et al. Guidance for pediatric end-of-life care. *Pediatrics.* 2022;149(5):e2022057011. doi:10.1542/peds.2022-057011.

20. Solis RN, Farber NI, Fairman N, et al. Bereavement practices among head and neck cancer surgeons. *Laryngoscope.* 2022;132(10):1971-1975. doi:10.1002/lary.30037.

21. Kusano AS, Kenworthy-Heinige T, Thomas CR Jr. Survey of bereavement practices of cancer care and palliative care physicians in the Pacific Northwest United States. *J Oncol Pract.* 2012;8(5):275-281. doi:10.1200/JOP.2011.000512.

22. Morris SE, Block SD. Adding value to palliative care services: The development of an institutional bereavement program. *J Palliat Med.* 2015;18(11):915-922. doi:10.1089/jpm.2015.0080.

23. Hufford D, Bucklin MA. The spirit of spiritual healing in the United States. In Koss-Chioino, Joan; Hefner, Philip (eds.). *Spiritual Transformation and Healing: Anthropological, Theological, Neuroscientific, and Clinical Perspectives.* Lanham, MD: AltaMira Press; 2005.

24. Greyson, B. *After: A Doctor Explores What Near-Death Experiences Reveal about Life and Beyond.* New York, NY: St. Martin's Essentials; 2021.

25. Jackson LL. *Signs: The Secret Language of the Universe.* New York, NY: Dial Press; 2020.

26. Tartaglia A, White KB, Corson T, et al. Supporting staff: The role of health care chaplains *J Health Care Chaplain.* 2022;1-14. doi:10.1080/08854726.2022.2154107.

Chapter 11

1. Rosenbaum E, Gordon AE, Cresta J, Shaughnessy AF, Jonas WB. Implementing whole person primary care: results from a year-long learning collaborative. *J Am Board Fam Med.* 2023 Aug 9;36(4):542-549. doi:10.3122/jabfm.2023.230007R1

2. Hui D, Bruera E. The Edmonton Symptom Assessment System 25 years later: past, present, and future developments. *J Pain Symptom Manage.* 2017;53(3):630-643. doi:10.1016/j.jpainsymman.2016.10.370.

3. American Institute for Cancer Research. Setting a SMART goal for AICR's recommendations. 2018. https://www.aicr.org/resources/blog/setting-a-smart-goal-to-meet-aicrs-physical-activity-recommendations/. Accessed August 31, 2023.

Chapter 12

1. Antonelli M, Donelli D, Barbieri G, et al. Forest volatile organic compounds and their effects on human health: A state-of-the-art review. *Int. J. Environ. Res. Public Health.* 2020; 17:6506.

2. Ulrich RS. View through a window may influence recovery from surgery. *Science.* 1984;224(4647):420-421. doi:10.1126/science.6143402.

3. Schneider CM, Hsieh CC, Sprod LK, Carter SD, Hayward R. Exercise training manages cardiopulmonary function and fatigue during and following cancer treatment in male cancer survivors. *Integr Cancer Ther.* 2007;6(3): 235-41.

4. Repka CP, Hayward R. Oxidative stress and fitness changes in cancer patients after exercise training. *Med Sci Sports Exerc.* 2016; 48(4): 607-14.

5. Knobf MT, Musanti R, Dorward J. Exercise and quality of life outcomes in patients with cancer. *Semin Oncol Nurs.* 2007; 23(4):285-96.

6. Bremer BA, Moore CT, Bourbon BM, Hess DR, Bremer KL. Perceptions of control, physical exercise, and psychological adjustment to breast cancer in South African women. *Ann Behav Med.* 1997;19(1):51-60. DOI: 10.1007/bf02883427.

7. Rock CL, Thomson C, Gansler T, Gapstur SM, McCullough ML, et al. American Cancer Society guideline for diet and physical activity for cancer prevention. *CA A Cancer J Clin.* 2020;70:245-271. doi.org/10.3322/caac.21591.

8. American College of Sports Medicine. Guidelines for Exercise and Cancer. www.ascm.org. Accessed August 31, 2023.

9. Crowley J, Ball L, Hiddink GJ. Nutrition in medical education: A systematic review. *Lancet Planet Health.* 2019 Sep;3(9):e379-e389. doi: 10.1016/S2542-5196(19)30171-8.

10. Samueli Foundation. US Patient & Oncologist Awareness, Usage, & Attitudes Toward Whole Person Integrative Oncology. Final Report: September 30, 2022 (Update Oct 7); Prepared for Samueli Foundation by IQVIA; healingworksfoundation.org/wp-content/uploads/2022/10/Samueli_Integrative-Oncology-Tracking-W1_Final-Report_7-Oct-2022.pdf. Access August 31, 2023.

11. Key TJ, Bradbury KE, Perez-Cornago A, et al. Diet, nutrition, and cancer risk: What do we know and what is the way forward? *BMJ.* 2020; 368:m511. doi.org/10.1136/bmj.m511.

12. Rowles JL, Erdman JW. Carotenoids and their role in cancer prevention. Bioch Biophy Act. 2020;1865(11):158613. doi:10.1016/j.bbalip.

2020.158613. Abdull Razis AF, Noor NM. Cruciferous vegetables: dietary phytochemicals for cancer prevention. *Asian Pac J Cancer Prev.* 2013;14(3):1565-70. doi: 10.7314/apjcp.2013.14.3.1565.

13. Schwingshackl L, Schwedhelm C, Galbete C, Hoffmann G. Adherence to Mediterranean diet and risk of cancer: An updated systematic review and meta-analysis. *Nutrients.* 2017 Sept 26;9(10):1063. doi:10.3390/nu9101063 .

14. Toledo E, Salas-Salvadó J, Donat-Vargas C, et al. Mediterranean diet and invasive breast cancer risk among women at high cardiovascular risk in the PREDIMED Trial: A randomized clinical trial. *JAMA Intern Med.* 2015;175(11):1752–1760. doi:10.1001/jamainternmed.2015.4838.

15. Katz R, Edelson M. *The Cancer-Fighting Kitchen.* Berkley, CA: Ten Speed Press; 2017.

16. PDQ® Supportive and Palliative Care Editorial Board. PDQ Nutrition in Cancer Care. Bethesda, MD: National Cancer Institute. https://www.cancer.gov/about-cancer/treatment/side-effects/appetite-loss/nutri-tion-pdq. Accessed August 31, 2023.

17. Ben-Arye E, Halabi I, Attias S, Goldstein L, Schiff E. Asking patients the right questions about herbal and dietary supplements: Cross cultural perspectives. *Complement Ther Med.* 2014;22(2):304-310. doi:10.1016/j.ctim.2014.01.005.

18. Meyer F, Bairati I, Fortin A, et al. Interaction between antioxidant vitamin supplementation and cigarette smoking during radiation therapy in relation to long-term effects on recurrence and mortality: A randomized trial among head and neck cancer patients. *Int J Cancer.* 2008;122(7):1679-1683. doi:10.1002/ijc.23200.

19. Klein EA, Thompson IM Jr, Tangen CM, et al. Vitamin E and the risk of prostate cancer: the Selenium and Vitamin E Cancer Prevention Trial (SELECT). *JAMA.* 2011;306(14):1549-1556. doi:10.1001/jama.2011.1437.

20. Savard J, Ivers H, Villa J, Caplette-Gingras A, Morin CM. Natural course of insomnia comorbid with cancer: an 18-month longitudinal study. *J Clin Oncol.* 2011 Sep 10;29(26):3580-6. doi: 10.1200/JCO.2010.33.2247.

21. Bean HR, Diggens J, Ftanou M, et al. Light enhanced cognitive behavioral therapy for insomnia and fatigue during chemotherapy for breast cancer: A randomized controlled trial. *Sleep.* 2022;45(3):zsab246. doi:10.1093/sleep/zsab246.

22. Shechter A, Kim EW, St-Onge MP, Westwood AJ. Blocking nocturnal blue light for insomnia: A randomized controlled trial. *J Psych Researh.* 2018; 96:196–202.

23. Kuhathasan N, Dufort A, MacKillop J, Gottschalk R, Minuzzi L, Frey BN. The use of cannabinoids for sleep: A critical review on clinical trials. *Exp Clin Psychopharmacol.* 2019;27(4):383-401. doi:10.1037/pha0000285.

24. Taha T, Meiri D, Talhamy S, et al. New drug development and clinical pharmacology cannabis impacts tumor response rate to nivolumab in patients with advanced malignancies. *Oncologist.* 2019; 24: 549–554.

25. La Marca L, Maniscalco E, Fabbiano F, Verderame F, Schimmenti A. Efficacy of Pennebaker's expressive writing intervention in reducing psychiatric symptoms among patients with first-time cancer diagnosis: a randomized clinical trial. *Support Care Cancer.* 2019;27(5):1801-1809. doi:10.1007/s00520-018-4438-0.

26. Jans-Beken L, Jacobs N, Janssens M. Gratitude and health: An updated review. *J Posit Psychol* 2020; 15(6):743-782. DOI: 10.1080/17439760.20 19.1651888.

27. PDQ® Supportive and Palliative Care Editorial Board. *PDQ Cancer-Related Post-Traumatic Stress.* Bethesda, MD: National Cancer Institute. https://www.cancer.gov/about-cancer/coping/survivorship/new-normal/ptsd-hp-pdq. Accessed August 31, 2023.

28. Gordon JS. *Transforming Trauma: The Path to Hope and Healing.* New York, NY: HarperOne; 2019.

29. Puchalski CM. The role of spirituality in health care. *Proc (Bayl Univ Med Cent).* 2001;14(4):352-357. doi:10.1080/08998280.2001.11927788.

30. Samueli Foundation. US patient & oncologist awareness, usage, & attitudes toward whole person integrative oncology final report, September 30, 2022 (update Oct 7).

31. Ripamonti CI, Giuntoli F, Gonella S, Miccinesi G. Spiritual care in cancer patients: A need or an option? *Curr Opin Oncol.* 2018;30(4):212-218. doi:10.1097/CCO.0000000000000454.

32. Wang YC, Lin CC. Spiritual well-being may reduce the negative impacts of cancer symptoms on the quality of life and the desire for hastened death in terminally ill cancer patients. *Cancer Nurs.* 2016;39(4):E43-E50. doi:10.1097/NCC.0000000000000298.

33. King DE, Bushwick B. Beliefs and attitudes of hospital inpatients about faith healing and prayer. *J Fam Pract.* 1994;39(4):349-352.

34. Damen A, Labuschagne D, Fosler L, et al. What do chaplains do: The views of palliative care physicians, nurses, and social workers. *Am J Hosp Palliat Care.* 2019;36(5):396-401. doi:10.1177/1049909118807123.

35. Borneman T, Ferrell B, Puchalski CM. Evaluation of the FICA tool for spiritual assessment. *J Pain Symptom Manage.* 2010;40(2):163-173. doi:10.1016/j.jpainsymman.2009.12.019.

36. Dossey L. *Healing Words: The Power of Prayer and the Practice of Medicine.* New York, NY: Harper One; 1995.

Chapter 13

1. Gao P, Gao XI, Fu T, Xu D, Wen Q. Acupuncture: Emerging evidence for its use as an analgesic (review). *Exp Ther Med.* 2015;9(5):1577-1581. doi:10.3892/etm.2015.2348. Ma Q. Somato-Autonomic Reflexes of Acupuncture. *Med Acupunct.* 2020;32(6):362-366. doi:10.1089/acu.2020.1488.

2. Hershman DL, Unger JM, Greenlee H, et al. Effect of acupuncture vs sham acupuncture or waitlist control on joint pain related to aromatase inhibitors among women with early-stage breast cancer: A randomized clinical trial. *JAMA.* 2018;320(2):167-176. doi:10.1001/jama.2018.8907.

3. Levy CE, Casler N, FitzGerald DB. Battlefield acupuncture: An emerging method for easing pain. *Am J Phys Med Rehabil.* 2018 Mar;97(3):e18-e19. doi: 10.1097/PHM.0000000000000766.

4. Wood MJ, Molassiotis A, Payne S. What research evidence is there for the use of art therapy in the management of symptoms in adults with cancer? A systematic review. *Psychooncology.* 2011;20(2):135-145. doi:10.1002/pon.1722.

5. Gramaglia C, Gambaro E, Vecchi C, et al. Outcomes of music therapy interventions in cancer patients-A review of the literature. *Crit Rev Oncol Hematol.* 2019;138:241-254.

6. Bradt J, Potvin N, Kesslick A, et al. The impact of music therapy versus music medicine on psychological outcomes and pain in cancer patients: a mixed methods study. *Support Care Cancer.* 2015;23(5):1261-1271. doi:10.1007/s00520-014-2478-7.

7. Bradt J, Dileo C, Myers-Coffman K, Biondo J. Music interventions for improving psychological and physical outcomes in people with cancer. *Cochrane Database Syst Rev.* 2021 Oct 12;10(10):CD006911. doi: 10.1002/14651858.CD006911.pub4.

8. Access to Care in Cancer: The Patient Experience. Survey results. Cancer Support Community. 2016. Accessed August 31, 2023.

9. Ramsey SD, Bansal A, Fedorenko CR, et al. Financial insolvency as a risk factor for early mortality among patients with cancer. *J Clin Oncol.* 2016;34(9):980-986. doi:10.1200/JCO.2015.64.6620.

10. Pan YQ, Yang KH, Wang YL, Zhang LP, Liang HQ. Massage interventions and treatment-related side effects of breast cancer: A systematic review and meta-analysis. *Int J Clin Oncol.* 2014;19(5):829-841. doi:10.1007/s10147-013-0635-5.

11. Müller M, Klingberg K, Wertli MM, Carreira H. Manual lymphatic drainage and quality of life in patients with lymphoedema and mixed oedema: a systematic review of randomised controlled trials. *Qual Life Res.* 2018 Jun;27(6):1403-1414. doi: 10.1007/s11136-018-1796-5.

12. Yao C, Cheng Y, Zhu Q, Lv Z, Kong L, Fang M. clinical evidence for the effects of manual therapy on cancer pain: A systematic review and meta-analysis. *Evid Based Complement Alternat Med.* 2021 Feb 5;2021:6678184. doi:10.1155/2021/6678184.

13. Qaseem A, Wilt TJ, McLean RM, Forciea MA. Noninvasive treatments for acute, subacute, and chronic low back pain: A clinical practice guideline from the American College of Physicians. *Ann Intern Med.* 2017;166(7):514- 530.

14. Gordon JS. Mind-body medicine and cancer. *Hem Onc Clin N Am.* 2008;22:683-708. https://doi.org/10.1016/j.hoc.2008.04.010.

15. Daniels S. Cognitive behavior therapy for patients with cancer. *J Adv Pract Oncol*. 2015 Jan-Feb;6(1):54-6.

16. Melton L. Cognitive behavioral therapy for sleep in cancer patients: Research, techniques, and individual considerations. *J Adv Pract Oncol*. 2018;9(7):732-740.

17. Lang-Rollin I, Berberich G. Psycho-oncology. *Dialogues Clin Neurosci*. 2018 Mar;20(1):13-22. doi: 10.31887/DCNS.2018.20.1/ilangrollin.

18. Kestenbaum A, McEniry KA, Friedman S, et al. Spiritual AIM: Assessment and documentation of spiritual needs in patients with cancer. *J Health Care Chaplain*. 2022;28(4):566-577. doi:10.1080/0885472 6.2021.2008170.

19. Damen A, Labuschagne D, Fosler L, et al. What do chaplains do: The views of palliative care physicians, nurses, and social workers. *Am J Hosp Palliat Care*. 2019;36(5):396-401. doi:10.1177/1049909118807123.

20. Jain S, Hammerschlag R, Mills P, et al. Clinical studies of biofield therapies: Summary, methodological challenges, and recommendations. *Glob Adv Health Med*. 2015;4(Suppl):58-66. doi:10.7453/gahmj.2015.034.suppl.

21. Carlson LE, Toivonen K, Flynn M, et al. The role of hypnosis in cancer care. *Curr Oncol Rep*. 2018 Nov 13;20(12):93. doi:10.1007/s11912-018-0739-1.

22. Ignoffo RJ, Knapp KK, Seung A, et al. Trends in the delivery of care to oncology patients in the United States: Emphasis on the role pharmacists on the healthcare team. *J Oncol Pharm Pract*. 2021;27(1):5-13. doi:10.1177/1078155220907674.

23. Ameri A, Salmanizadeh F, Bahaadinbeigy K. Tele-pharmacy: A new opportunity for consultation during the COVID-19 pandemic. *Health Policy Technol*. 2020;9(3):281-282. doi:10.1016/j.hlpt.2020.06.005.

24. Brennan L, Sheill G, O'Neill L, et al. Physical therapists in oncology settings: Experiences in delivering cancer rehabilitation services, barriers to care, and service development needs. *Phys Ther*. 2022 Mar 1;102(3):pzab287. doi: 10.1093/ptj/pzab287.

25. Klein I, Kalichman L, Chen N, Susmallian S. A pilot study evaluating the effect of early physical therapy on pain and disabilities after breast cancer surgery: Prospective randomized control trail. *Breast*. 2021;59:286-293. doi:10.1016/j.breast.2021.07.013.

26. Campbell KL, Winters-Stone KM, Schmitz KH. We all seem to agree: Exercise is medicine in medical oncology. *J Clin Oncol*. 2023;41(1):147-148. doi:10.1200/JCO.22.01448.

27. Woodyard C. Exploring the therapeutic effects of yoga and its ability to increase quality of life. *Int J Yoga*. 2011;4(2):49-54.

28. Enfield S. Why more western doctors are now prescribing yoga therapy. *Yoga Journal*. February 3, 2016. Accessed August 31, 2023.

29. Woodyard C. Exploring the therapeutic effects of yoga and its ability to increase quality of life. *Int J Yoga*. 2011;4(2):49-54.

30. Cohen L, Warneke C, Fouladi RT, Rodriguez MA, Chaoul-Reich A. Psychological adjustment and sleep quality in a randomized trial of the effects of a Tibetan yoga intervention in patients with lymphoma. *Cancer.* 2004;100(10):2253-2260.

31. XiangY, Lu L, Chen X, Wen Z. Does Tai Chi relieve fatigue? A systematic review and meta-analysis of randomized controlled trials. *PLoS One 2017; 12*(4): e0174872.

32. Zeng Y, Luo T, Xie H, Huang M, Cheng AS. Health benefits of qigong or tai chi for cancer patients: A systematic review and meta-analyses. *Complement Ther Med.* 2014;22(1):173-86.

Chapter 14

1. Access to Care in Cancer: The Patient Experience. Survey results. Cancer Support Community. 2016. Accessed August 31, 2023.

2. Mao JJ, Palmer CS, Healy KE, Desai K, Amsterdam J. Complementary and alternative medicine use among cancer survivors: a population-based study. *J Cancer Surviv.* 2011 Mar;5(1):8-17. doi: 10.1007/s11764-010-0153-7.

3. Crudup T. Whole-person integrative oncology–A path to improved outcomes and patient empowerment. Open Access Government. January 2023;80-81. doi.org/10.56367/OAG-037-10637.

4. Samueli Foundation. US Patient & Oncologist Awareness, Usage, & Attitudes Toward Whole Person Integrative Oncology. Final Report: September 30, 2022 (Update Oct 7); Prepared for Samueli Foundation by IQVIA; healingworksfoundation.org/wp-content/uploads/2022/10/Samueli_Integrative-Oncology-Tracking-W1_Final-Report_7-Oct-2022.pdf. Access August 31, 2023.

5. Bari S, Chineke I, Darwin A, Umar A, Jim H, Muzaffar J, Singh S, Kucuk O. Awareness, use and outlook of complementary and alternative medicine (CAM) options in an underserved, uninsured minority cancer patient population. [Erratum in: *Integr Cancer Ther.* 2022 Jan-Dec;21:15347354221076921.] *Integr Cancer Ther.* 2021 Jan-Dec;20:15347354211051622. doi: 10.1177/15347354211051622.

6. Karim S, Benn R, Carlson LE, et al. integrative oncology education: An emerging competency for oncology providers. *Curr Oncol.* 2021 Feb 10;28(1):853-862. doi: 10.3390/curroncol28010084.

7. Abrams DI. *Integrative Oncology.* (eds) Weil A. New York, NY: Oxford University Press, 2nd ed; 2014.

8. Veterans Administration, Health Services Research & Development, Evidence Synthesis Program Reports. https://hsrd.research.va.gov/publications/esp/reports.cfm. Accessed August 31, 2023.

9. Veterans Administration, Health Services Research & Development, Evidence Map: Acupuncture as Treatment for Adult Health Conditions (Update from 2013 - 2021), https://hsrd.research.va.gov/publications/esp/acupuncture-evidence-map.cfm. Accessed August 31, 2023.

10. Society for Integrative Oncology, Practice Guidelines. integrativeonc. org/practice-guidelines/guidelines. Accessed August 31, 2023.

11. Hershman DL, Unger JM, Greenlee H, et al: Effect of acupuncture vs sham acupuncture or waitlist control on joint pain related to aromatase inhibitors among women with early-stage breast cancer: A randomized clinical trial. *JAMA*. 2018; 320:167-176.

12. Deng GE, Rausch SM, Jones LW, et al. Complementary therapies and integrative medicine in lung cancer: diagnosis and management of lung cancer, 3rd ed: American College of Chest Physicians evidence-based clinical practice guidelines. *Chest*. 2013;143(Suppl 5):e420S-36S.

13. Ng JY, Nault H, Nazir Z. Complementary and integrative medicine mention and recommendations: A systematic review and quality assessment of lung cancer clinical practice guidelines. *Integr Med Res*. 2021 Mar;10(1):100452. doi: 10.1016/j.imr.2020.100452.

14. Shani P, Walter E. Acceptability and use of mind-body interventions among African American cancer survivors: An integrative review. *Integr Cancer Ther*. 2022 Jan-Dec;21:15347354221103275. doi: 10.1177/15347354221103275.

15. Worster B, Hajjar ER, Handley N. Cannabis use in patients with cancer: A clinical review. *JCO Oncol Pract*. 2022;18(11):743-749. doi:10.1200/ OP.22.00080.

16. Campbell KL, Winters-Stone KM, Wiskemann J, et al. exercise guidelines for cancer survivors: consensus statement from international multidisciplinary roundtable. *Med Sci Sports Exerc*. 2019;51(11):2375-2390. doi:10.1249/MSS.0000000000002116.

17. Ligibel JA, Bohlke K, May AM, et al. Exercise, diet, and weight management during cancer treatment: ASCO Guideline. *J Clin Oncol*. 2022;40(22):2491-2507. doi:10.1200/JCO.22.00687.

18. Centers for Medicare & Medicaid Services. Enhancing oncology model. https://innovation.cms.gov/innovation-models/enhancing-oncology-model. Accessed August 31. 2023.

19. National Cancer Institute. Financial toxicity and cancer treatment. cancer.gov/about-cancer/managing-care/track-care-costs/financial-toxicity-hp-pdq#_94_toc. Accessed August 31, 2023.

20. Institute of Medicine and National Research Council. 2006. *From Cancer Patient to Cancer Survivor: Lost in Transition*. Washington, DC: The National Academies Press. https://doi.org/10.17226/11468.

21. Institute of Medicine. 2013. *Delivering High-Quality Cancer Care: Charting a New Course for a System in Crisis*. Washington, DC: The National Academies Press. https://doi.org/10.17226/18359

22. National Academies of Sciences, Engineering, and Medicine. 2023. *Achieving Whole Health: A New Approach for Veterans and the Nation*. Washington, DC: The National Academies Press. https://doi. org/10.17226/26854.

Chapter 15

1. Sakallaris BR, MacAllister L, Voss M, Smith K, Jonas WB. Optimal healing environments. *Glob Adv Health Med.* 2015;4(3):40-45. doi:10.7453/gahmj.2015.043.

2. Christianson J, Finch M, Findlay B, Goertz C, Jonas WB. *Reinventing the Patient Experience: Strategies for Hospital Leaders.* Chicago, IL: Health Administration Press; 2007. Ananth S, Jonas WB. Implementing OHE's. *Explore.* 2010;6(1):52-53.

3. Jonas WB, Rosenbaum E. The case for whole-person integrative care. *Medicina (Kaunas).* 2021 June 30;57(7):677. doi:10.3390/medicina57070677.

4. Bokhour BG, Hyde J, Kligler B, et al. From patient outcomes to system change: Evaluating the impact of VHA's implementation of the Whole Health System of Care. *Health Serv Res.* 2022;57(Suppl 1):53-65. doi:10.1111/1475-6773.13938.

5. US Department of Veterans Affairs. Whole System Health Care Evaluation. https://www.va.gov/WHOLEHEALTH/docs/EPCC_WHS evaluation_FinalReport_508.pdf. Accessed August 31, 2023.

6. National Academies of Sciences, Engineering, and Medicine. 2023. *Achieving whole health: A new approach for veterans and the nation.* Washington, DC: The National Academies Press. https://doi.org/10.17226/26854.

7. Institute for Healthcare Improvement. Quality improvement essentials toolkit. https://www.ihi.org/resources/Pages/Tools/Quality-Improvement-Essentials-Toolkit.aspx. Accessed August 31, 2023.

8. US Department of Veterans Affairs. Creating options for Veterans' expedited recovery. Final report. https://www.va.gov/COVER/docs/COVER-Commission-Final-Report-2020-01-24.pdf. January 24, 2020. Accessed August 31, 2023.

9. Porter ME, Lee TH. Integrated practice units: A playbook for health care leaders. *NEJM Catal Innov Care Deliv.* 2021;2(1). DOI: 10.1056/CAT.20.0237.

10. Leaf C. *The Truth in Small Doses: Why We're Losing the War on Cancer—and How to Win It.* New York, NY: Simon & Schuster; 2014.

11. Jonas WB, Adibe B. An integrated framework for achieving national health goals. *JAMA Health Forum.* 2022;3(5):e221109. doi:10.1001/jamahealthforum.2022.1109.

12. The Samueli Institute at the Davidoff Center: Towards the Next Breakthrough in Cancer. https://hospitals.clalit.co.il/rabin/en/departments/cancer_davidoff_center/Pages/the_samueli_institute.aspx. Accessed August 31, 2023.

13. Jamaica Hospital Medical Center. Patient Centered Care. https://jamaicahospital.org/patient-services/person-centered-care/. Accessed August 31, 2023.

14. Osarogiagbon RU, Rodriguez HP, Hicks D, et al. Deploying team science principles to optimize interdisciplinary lung cancer care delivery: Avoiding the long and winding road to optimal care. *J Oncol Pract.* 2016;12(11):983-991. Doi:10.1200/JOP.2016.013813.

15. Agency for Healthcare Research and Quality. Health Literacy Universal Precautions Toolkit, 2nd Edition. https://www.ahrq.gov/ health-literacy/improve/precautions/tool2b.html#:~:text=The%20 Plan%2DDo%2DStudy%2D,on%20it%2C%20and%20testing%20again. Accessed August 31. 2023.

FURTHER
INFORMATION

Visit the book website
HealingandCancerBook.com
for all the resources mentioned
in this book and more.

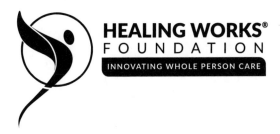

Healing Works Foundation's mission is to make whole person, integrative care regular and routine. Led by Dr. Wayne Jonas, HWF partners with a diverse group of wellbeing innovators. It creates platforms, processes, programs, tools and services to support and magnify insights and innovations in healing and whole person care principally in primary care and oncology.